There __Is__ a Cure
for
the Common Cold

There <u>Is</u> a Cure
for
the Common Cold

Edmé Régnier, M. D.

Parker Publishing Company Inc.
West Nyack, New York

© 1971 *by*

PARKER PUBLISHING COMPANY, INC.
West Nyack, New York

Library of Congress
Catalog Card Number: 72-160510

Printed in the United States of America
ISBN-0-13-914945-7
B & P

This book is dedicated to the
professional nursing staff
and the
technical, clerical, and
maintenance workers
of the
Josiah B. Thomas Hospital
Peabody, Massachusetts,
all of whom have been unfailingly
helpful to me for some twenty years

IMPORTANT

If you have a *brand new* cold right now—one not more than 24 hours old—please turn directly to the introduction for immediate help.

If your cold is more than a day old already, or if you have no cold at all at this time, it will be best for you to take the time *now* to read through the whole of this book carefully, so you can be fully ready to meet, and to *defeat* your *next* cold, when it appears, or better still, to prevent it from ever happening.

Introduction

Do you have a fresh cold right now? Here is help.

I strongly recommend that you do *not* treat yourself with vitamin C (ascorbic acid) for even one cold until you have read—and thoroughly *understood*—this book, at least all parts of it up to and including chapter 5.

I will make one exception to this. If you are sure you *already* know exactly what is meant by *every* term that is appearing in these paragraphs of this Introduction you are reading right now, and *if* your cold meets *all* the conditions I am going to put down here and now, then it will be safe for you to get started treating your cold within the next five minutes, to start getting with it right now. But for your own good, you must promise me that you will go on and read chapters 1 through 5 within the next six hours, by which time you will be just ready for your third dose of vitamin C. I never allow my own personal patients to go any further with vitamin C than this by themselves, until I have made certain they understand exactly what they are doing with this very powerful medicine. You deserve the same careful approach in this book. Following is an example of what I mean.

Mr. J.T., age 35, a salesman, using his excellently developed powers of persuasion, got past my secretary without an appointment, and hoarsely begged me:

"Doc, they say you can stop a cold like magic. I'm due in Detroit tomorrow for a conference at the home office. If it keeps going like this I'll have to *write* my report on a pad and *hand* it to the sales manager. Fix me up, will you?"

"How long have you had this cold now, Mr. T?" I asked. "When did it begin?"

"It came on Tuesday evening, Doc," he recounted. (This figured up to about 60 hours, some two and a half days ago.)

"I'm sorry, J.T.," I had to tell him. "You're too late this time. You have to get to it before that. If you tried vitamin C now, and it didn't work, which it probably wouldn't, you'd be discouraged, and I'd lose my best chance to get you in line for future colds. I'm sorry, but it's in your own best interest, believe me. How about making an appointment for when you get back, and we'll go over the whole thing? Tell my secretary I said not to charge you."

(He did return, and eventually became one of my strongest supporters.)

As for *your* cold, the one *you* have right now:

1. Have you had it less than 24 hours, measured back from right now? Are you sure you were perfectly all right at this same time yesterday, that you didn't have anything wrong yet at the time, and that you had no inkling then you were about to come down with a cold?
   (Your answers here must all be "Yes.")

2. Do you have some *fresh* vitamin C (any brand) in a *sealed* bottle that hasn't been opened at all yet?
   (Your answer must be "Yes.")

3. Do you understand exactly what is meant by so and so many "milligrams" of vitamin C? Do you recognize what that term means as to the size of the dose of the medicine that you will be taking?
   (Your answer must be "Yes.")

4. Have you eaten any large amount (more than ½ pint) of either yogurt or buttermilk in the past 8 hours?
   (Your answer to this one must be "No.")

5. You're pretty sure this *is* a cold, the kind of thing *you* have when you have a cold, aren't you?
   (Your answer must be "Yes.")

If *all* your answers are the correct ones, all "Yes" but #4, and that one "No," then immediately take 750 mg. of your freshly opened vitamin C, right now, by swallowing of course, with any amount of water you need to take it down. If it's mealtime just about now, eat relatively little to give this first dose of vitamin C a better chance to start absorbing into your system. This light eating is not very important after the first couple of doses. Your next dose of vitamin C will be due in three hours (to an accuracy of five or ten minutes one way or the other, but no more leeway) and it will then be 625 mg. Take it at the proper time.

Please begin reading the first five chapters of this book, through chapter 5, and finish up within the next six hours, at which time you will be taking your third dose, again 625 mg. By this time you will have learned a lot more than you probably know now about colds. Your next specific directions for your fourth dose and all succeeding doses will be coming from chapter 5.

Don't expect *any* good result at all to show itself just yet. You have to have been on the medicine for about 12 to 18 hours before you'll notice improvement. It takes that long to start any real cold control that you can appreciate. Once you have put in that much time you will begin to be quite pleased with yourself to say the least.

Edmé Régnier, M. D.

The basic scientific research which underlies the recommendations in this book was presented to the medical profession in the professional medical journal *Review of Allergy*, September and October 1968 issues.

To physicians. the reference is—

Régnier, E.: The Administration of Large Doses of Ascorbic Acid in the Prevention and Treatment of the Common Cold, Parts I and II, *Review of Allergy:* 22: 835, 948 (1968).

Contents

Chapter 2 (continued)

**Chapter   3 . . . . . . .What You Should Know
                        About Vitamin C. 39**

Chapter 5 (continued)

Chapter 5 (continued)

Chapter 5 (continued)

There Is a Cure
for
the Common Cold

1

You Can Do Something About Your Cold

Must you John, or you, Mary, or more to the point, *you* who are reading this right now, whatever your name may be, *must* you patiently submit to whatever miseries a cold chooses to inflict upon you? Regardless of what you may have thought up to now, the answer to this question is, positively, "No, you don't have to take that kind of punishment from a cold." You ask, "You mean to tell me I *don't* have to just take whatever a cold cares to dump on me, and not be able to really do anything about it?" My answer to that is, again, "No, you needn't take it. You don't have to go through those miseries if you choose not to. The choice is yours."

It is no longer necessary for you to take the insults of a cold lying down—and it may interest you to know that it hasn't *been* necessary for about the past 15 to 20 years. That's about how long ago at least a few people—a handful of doctors, and a lot more of the public at large, incidentally—began to catch on to what vitamin C could really do against that recurring, all-too-familiar annoyance, the common cold, or as we call it for short, just "a cold."

"All right, *what* will it do?" you ask, "What can vitamin C do for *me* and *my* cold? What's in it for me?"

I'll tell you what it can do for you. *All* of the following, not just one of these things.

25

WHAT VITAMIN C CAN DO FOR YOUR COLD

(1) It can make it considerably less likely that you will catch any cold at all—the year round.

(2) It can make any cold that you do catch a "smaller" cold than it would otherwise be—a shorter and less serious one.

(3) It can protect you from catching a cold from a particular person whom you can see obviously has a cold, but whom you're unable to avoid, such as someone who coughs near you, or suddenly sneezes in your vicinity.

(4) It can so powerfully keep under control any cold that you have been unlucky enough to catch a good hold on, that you will not be put out of commission for a single moment. You will be able to go right on with your ordinary life without any of the usual miseries of a cold—not a single one of them.

No runny nose! (Remember that itchy drip sliding slowly down the inside of your nose? How could your forget it? How about the raw, burned skin around your nostrils?) No stuffiness. ("Am I *ever* sick of having to keep my mouth open to breathe!") No sore throat. No hoarseness. No sneezing. No cough. No loss of taste. ("Mildred, did you make this dish out of cardboard?") No malaise—what doctors call the feeling of being sick. ("Boy, do I feel lousy!")

YOU DON'T HAVE TO CATCH A COLD

You don't have to put up with *any* annoyances of a cold if you don't want to. The *right* amount of vitamin C taken at the *right* time can spare you many an uncomfortable moment. Our enemy the common cold *can* be held in check very nicely, and very nearly all the time. Anyone who's gone through the pleasures of having colds in the past—and that, of course, is practically all of us—finds vitamin C's powers to hold a cold in check truly amazing, nothing less than remarkable. This goes whether you already have a cold—and have it under control—or just don't want to get one.

The Case of Harriet B.

Mrs. Harriet B., a not-so-young member of the "Thread and Needles" Sewing Society, sidled up to me at a reception. "Sally tells me," she "zeroed" in on me, "that you could see to it that I didn't have a cold on the evening of Thursday, February 15." (Some eight weeks off.)

"I have wanted to see a certain New York show for months now, but it's so hard to get a ticket. Now, I can finally get one, but I don't want to promise to go down to New York at a specific time in the future, especially during a month like February, with the hotel reservations and all that, and then have a cold spoil it all!"

How You Can Hold a Cold in Check

The upshot of it was that Mrs. B. came over to the office, satisfied me she meant business, and quickly mastered the Simple Art of Vitamin C. Sure enough, exactly two evenings before her tickets and reservations in the Big City she came down with a nice cold—which she allowed to run just about the 15 hours it took her to be sure it was for real. She took off as scheduled, her cold held in excellent check by vitamin C.

Your own tastes may not run to stage shows, but you can be equally certain of turning up at hockey playoffs, and in the good voice you'll need to express your opinions of that visiting goalie. I hope you're lucky enough not to have a cold when you get to the hockey arena, even though you could be mastering it nicely with vitamin C, if necessary. But the question is, if you haven't got a cold when you get there, will you have one when you leave? You don't *have* to run the slightest risk of picking up a cold from the crowds of coughers!

You can be royalty, you can be a prince, no, far better than that, *you* can be the charmed one, *you* may walk untouched among the touched—the touched by colds, that is. *They* may have their colds, but they're not going to hand them to you, because they don't know what *you* know, as I will tell you now.

YOU DON'T HAVE TO SPREAD A COLD

One other nice thing that vitamin C can do for you and your cold, I don't say that it's necessarily the best of all, but Susan L., who was one of the original "testers" in my early research in treating colds, had no question in *her* mind:

"Doctor, the best thing about this whole vitamin C thing is that I don't give my cold to the babies." (Two of them, ages two and three.) "Ever since Don and I have been coming over here (my office) *we* haven't given a cold to either of them."

A cold that is held in check by vitamin C treatment cannot easily be transmitted to someone else. That is a very big plus.

THE THREE BASICS OF BEATING A COLD

There are only three things you need to give yourself a really remarkable power over your own fate when you meet up with a cold, over what happens to you in that situation. All three things are absolutely necessary. None of them can be missing. *First,* you need vitamin C. *Second,* you need your own good judgment, intelligence, and determination to succeed. This is the *most* important one of the three things you need. *Finally,* you need the *instructions* on how to use vitamin C. As far as I know, the complete instructions, written in simple language, are available *nowhere in the world at this time except within the covers of this one book you are reading.* I myself am the physician who developed the instructions, based largely on my own medical research, and taking into consideration the work of other doctors in the past, and the experiences of thousands of the general public over the past 30 years. As is the custom in medical science, this material has first been presented in technical form to the medical profession in scientific reports for their prior approval, several years ago. Now it is being presented for the first time to the public at large. This book *is* the set of instructions and programs *you* will need to use vitamin C to conquer your colds.

2

Understanding Is the Key to Your Power Over the Common Cold

About thirty years ago I had one big problem. I was at the age when my one big problem, if any, should have been girls, I guess. It wasn't. Except for the three months of June, July, and August of each summer, I lived in horror of my own personal, long-established bogeyman, *the common cold,* and what it would surely do to me at our next encounter. I used to dread the coming of fall, even though that lovely season brought the autumnal leaves skittering across the sidewalks.

THE ANNUAL BEGINNING OF MY COLD MISERIES

With October, and sometimes even with September, was sure to come my first glorious cold of the season, inevitably to "settle" into my ears. That meant a beginning at about midnight of such torturing pressure on my eardrums (structures magnificently supplied with *three different* sets of super-sensitive nerves) that I had to walk the dark streets for hours to make the pain seem a little less—a little less in comparison with all the sounds and sights and smells of the city at night. For a time I kept a sizable jug of cod liver oil stashed on the window sill of my dorm room, where it would stay a little cooler, and taste, hopefully, a little less nauseating. When I got the beginning roughness in my throat that always meant the cold would succeed in climbing into my ears within a few short hours, I'd take down 22 tablespoons of cod liver oil. What did it do for me? Nothing. Nothing, period.

Cod Liver Oil Had the Wrong Vitamin for Me

Believe me, there was nothing even mildly amusing about all this at the time, to me. But now, many safe years later, now that I am absolute Master of the common cold, it does amuse me a little to think just how close I had been to the answer, hovering somewhere near it, yet unable to grab on to what would have spared me so many hours of misery still to come. I was toying about with a *vitamin,* yes, but unfortunately it wasn't the *right* vitamin. Cod liver oil is very, very rich in vitamin *A*. But vitamin *C* was what was really needed. As to that, at one point in those long ago days—of course I was to see this only many years later—I *was* pretty close to the right answer.

At the Lexington Market, then still a partly open-to-the-sky assemblage of vegetable and fruit stands, I bought myself 40 oranges. After cutting my roommate in for four of them, all he'd take, I proceeded to skin through and down the other 36 of them straight. That would have been enough vitamin C to put a notable halt into a cold not too far along, but at the time I didn't have any cold and was just gorging oranges because I liked them. I knew practically nothing about vitamin C then, I'd barely heard of it, and hadn't the faintest suspicion of what it could do. So my troubles with colds had some years to run yet.

OTHER MISERIES I EXPERIENCED

Over all, on at least 65 occasions all the way from the time I was a second-grade school kid of seven through the next 20 years every cold I ever had would stretch one or both, usually both, of my eardrums to the breaking point and make me the prisoner of a temporary deafness as well, for three to four weeks of near-silence at a time. This interference with my hearing, though it was dreadfully painful only the first several days, made it very hard for me to grasp the various lectures in medical school at times when I was going through one of my deaf periods. When I had grown up enough to start thinking carefully about these things, I had been somewhat surprised to notice that my ears, if they were going to "close," always did so only between the hours of 8 P.M. in the evening and midnight, always within that particular four hour stretch, and never within the other twenty hours of the day. (This, I was later to find out, was because the general resistance of my body to an infection by disease germs was naturally lowest at this particular portion of my own daily cycle. Everybody has similar periods of more or less resistance to germs in his own 24 hours of every day.)

By the age of 27 I had personally suffered through many different eras of treatment for colds and earaches, through many stages and various types of treatment for colds and the further disease complications that colds bring with them.

My earaches were one such complication. Such complications are "secondary," that is, following secondarily on the basic cold. They are usually caused not by the virus (a very tiny germ, we'll discuss this later) which caused the cold itself, but usually by bacteria (germs somewhat larger than viruses, and different in other ways, too). Complications of the common cold are bacteria germ involvements of such organs as the *lungs* (pneumonia). The back of the *throat* can also be invaded by bacteria in addition to the original cold viruses, and we call this complication "bacterial pharyngitis." Since the *tonsils* are in the pharynx, tonsillitis is really a part of pharyngitis. An infection of the voice box and vocal cords is called "laryngitis." Otitis, a germ infection of the *ears,* was of course my particular bugaboo, and it is a very common complication of a cold.

In the past, before we had penicillin and the sulfonamide medicines, otitis all too often led on further to mastoid trouble, wherein the infection had penetrated itself into the mastoid bone behind the ear. Sometimes there could be a still further step, the infection breaking out of the mastoid and on into the brain cavity, which complication is called "meningitis," or "brain abscess," depending on its exact location.

These complications have killed many a child, and they still are doing so in some places where modern medicine has been slow to reach. What a horrible succession of events—pharyngitis to otitis to mastoiditis to brain abscess to a hole in the ground, *and every bit of it based right back on that little cold so easily caught by an innocent youngster.*

It is possible to get these infections (germ diseases) in the ears, lungs, throat, sinuses, and trachea *without* having any cold preceding, that is, to have them caused by bacteria unaccompanied by cold viruses, in which case we can't call them a complication of a cold, but instead have to call them primary bacterial infections. However, the chances of having these organs invaded by bacteria germs are much greater if a cold is there first to "rough up" the protective surfaces of the tissues (flesh), which makes it easier for bacteria to attack them.

THE ANATOMY OF A COLD

You will notice that all these complications of a cold, all of these extra added attractions that the ordinary "plain" cold *usually* doesn't open the doorway to, but all too often does, are concerned with those structures of the body that are parts of what we call the "respiratory," that is, breathing, system. This is because the particular viruses that cause *colds* specifically "like" the respiratory system. That's the part of the body that these particular germs are "designed," you might say, to invade, enter, and live in, at least for a while.

The fact that you have a malaise, or ill-feeling, with a cold does not necessarily mean that the cold-causing viruses are themselves actually *in* the brain or some other part of the body *outside* their favorite part of the respiratory system. Probably they have caused some unpleasant chemical to be released into the blood stream, which can then affect the rest of the body at least to a minor degree. (Should it interest you, there *are* all sorts of other disease-causing viruses which, between them, *can* enter practically every corner of the body, even if the common cold viruses are pretty much restricted to the breathing passages.)

For 20 years in succession I was put through every treatment for colds and the secondary ear trouble, every treatment that a doting mother, a series of conscientious family doctors, and finally the expert specialists of one of the most famous medical school hospitals in the world knew anything about, or could think of. None of it did the slightest good for me.

THE USE OF VARIOUS "CURE-ALLS" TO NO AVAIL

Hot water bottles didn't do anything. "Cubeb" cigarette smoke blown in my ear by my mother, who never in her life smoked for any other purpose, gave no relief past the feeling of attention I was getting. Painting my throat with iodine felt good—for perhaps all of five minutes. A second removal of my adenoids at age 21 had no worthwhile result. A series of radium rays to the inside of my nose proved of no value either. Spraying my throat repeatedly with a strange solution called "sulfadiazine in triethylamine" (one of the first of the sulfa medicines, and now long discarded) had no useful effect. Long "baths" under the ultraviolet lamp neither cured nor prevented my colds.

For the first twenty years that I had frequent colds and earaches not a single thing that was ever tried to help me did me even the most minor good. Every bit of it was totally useless, except for what scant comfort I might be able to draw from the attention I was getting, which I hardly need tell you is not even worth the bother.

Yet for all of this time there existed a medicine that could easily have put an end to all my miseries. A medicine was readily available at every corner drug store in the country for very little money, and obtainable without even a prescription order from a doctor. A medicine that was sitting there waiting to help me many years before anybody had ever even heard of the word "penicillin," or ever dreamed that such a thing as "interferon" would ever be discovered. (*Don't* get the idea that I am saying penicillin is any good for a *cold;* it is *not,* but it is marvelous for some of the complications.) What I'm trying to make clear is that long ago we *already* had an excellent treatment for colds available, long before any of the recent discoveries. Some of these recent discoveries, like penicillin, can at least help some of the *complications* of colds (though not the basic cold), and one new finding at least, interferon, (given enough more time and a lot more special research work) may be able to do something for the cold itself, too. However, *right now* vitamin C can already do something— something good—against the basic cold.

THE SAD LACK OF KNOWLEDGE
OF VITAMIN C POSSIBILITIES

Why didn't I get vitamin C for my own long story of colds if it was there and waiting? Why did a fellow who didn't have just one cold one time, but had colds repeatedly—some 65 of them over a twenty year period—why didn't that fellow at least get *his* colds controlled by vitamin C, if it existed, and if it's as good as I say it is? Because *nobody* (or at least nobody I ran into) *knew* what vitamin C could do for colds. It was only *knowledge* that was missing, the knowledge to put together two already existing things—colds and vitamin C—together in the proper mix. What was needed was only a reshuffling of two already known things. No new materials or newly discovered ingredients were necessary, just brain power at work and more of it. More brain power was the difference between having had to go through what I went through and not having had to go through it. *Understanding* was all that was missing.

HOW TO EMANCIPATE YOURSELF FROM
THE CLUTCHES OF THE COMMON COLD

Now I believe you can see why I have asked you to listen to this long and sorry recital of my own history of unpleasant colds and more horrible earaches. It is not because I get any pleasure from the retelling of the story, but because I want to do everything I can to convince *you* of the absolute need for you to learn and thoroughly understand every fact about the common cold. *That* is what's going to make the difference between *you* and those others who will have to continue to suffer through igno- rantly with their colds. Your *knowledge* about colds will make the difference. Also, you must clearly understand everything we know about the workings of vitamin C as it goes about fighting a cold for you.

This is so because vitamin C will show its remarkable powers against colds only if it is being used exactly correctly. *It must be taken in sufficiently large quantities* (doses) and at very specific time intervals during the treatment. It must be begun *early* enough in a cold, and the strength of the doses must be adjusted in a very accurate way during the course of a cold. If it is to be used to *prevent* your catching a cold, rather than to treat one you already have, then it must be used according to one of several special programs for that particular purpose, which are different from the treatment plan. Equally important, if your chances of helping a particular cold are slim (usually this is one you started to treat too late) then you must not use vitamin C at all since you have practically no chance of success with it. This is because this is a *very* powerful medicine—when used in sizable doses. If it is *overused,* unnecessarily, to no useful purpose, it *does* have some capability of harming you. True, this is not a great deal of harm, but why risk *anything* for nothing?

Vitamin C *can* do something against colds that you will not believe possible until you have personally experienced it. It can hold a cold in suspended animation, allowing it to cause you no discomfort at all, until it has "burned itself out" and gone completely away. But getting vitamin C to do that, to do just exactly what you want it to do in a cold is a *rather critical* matter. It isn't anything you can be sloppy about. It isn't something you can be careless about—at least if you're going to take vitamin C in oral (pill) form, which is what I want you to do, rather than by needle injection. (Injection is not nearly as easy for you, and anyway isn't readily available to you at this time.)

WHY YOU MUST FOLLOW A STRICT PROGRAM

Unfortunately, a program for vitamin C that is somewhat carelessly carried out does not turn out to be at least some help in a cold; such a sloppy treatment course is usually *worthless* to you, and worse than that, it can be harmful. If *enough* vitamin C is taken sloppily—in a *poorly timed,* not well maintained schedule—it can make your cold drag on *longer* than it would ever have done if you had left it alone. A careless schedule will give you *no* useful relief either. Such an unsatisfactory performance usually results from taking doses of vitamin C that aren't *quite* large enough (though they may seem very large to some people)—or from taking doses that are spread too far apart, possibly just a little too far apart. (For the first five to six days of treating a cold with vitamin C, the doses must usually come every three hours, not further apart than that unless you are using long-acting vitamin C, or unless it's the one daily dose you're safely allowed to space out—the middle of the night one.

How to Avoid False Hopes About Vitamin C

The major reason why vitamin C has often failed to control colds for some people in the past is because they just didn't *know* what they were doing with it. They were stabbing in the dark, without clear knowledge of the amount of the medicine really needed or the timetable it has to be taken on. To these people vitamin C often proved to be just another false hope, another false lead in a long succession of false hopes that a really effective treatment for colds could be found. The actual fact is that vitamin C really does work successfully against colds with just about as great a success rate as any famous and well known medicine you could name succeeds in working against *its* special disease. Something like a 95 per cent success rate. That kind of a success record would be very good indeed for, say, penicillin when it is asked to work against the very "bugs" it's best suited to, in a disease such as pneumonia, for example.

Effective Vitamin C Program Easy to Follow

However, don't let me give you the idea for an instant that using vitamin C for a cold is going to be so difficult and complex that *you* won't be able to handle it. No such thing.

At about this point in one discussion, Bill cut into the talk with: "Doc, I never was no good at mathematics. I wonder if I can do this?"

Well, it was true that Bill hadn't hit it off in school as well as some others do, and it hadn't taken too much to get him to drop out of East High and then enlist in the Marines. Once in the service he'd been promptly assigned, and kept assigned exclusively, to the mothering of two and a half ton transport trucks. Very few people ever found out about his Purple Heart, I guess because he felt that being struck by a piece of enemy shrapnel while working in a motor pool, forward though it was, somehow wasn't very honorable. But back home again he'd gone to work with a local auto dealer as a tune-up expert.

"Bill," I assured him, "anybody who can stick an oh-twenty-two thousandth feeler gauge between the points inside a distributor can surely handle the arithmetic in this deal. There's nothing to it but keeping some sort of eye on the clock and being able to break a pill in half here, or add one pill to one pill to get a total of two pills there. The most important part of the whole set-up is just your own determination to make good on this job, the job of treating your cold."

Knowing what you're doing is absolutely vital if you want to put yourself into a better spot against the common cold. To avoid most colds, and to cut the others down to size, you must *know* the beast—know its tricks and understand the standard battle plans it will use against you. While you must never be afraid to turn and run from a cold, if you possibly can—that's the smart thing to do, avoid it if you can—you will sometimes *have* to stand and fight. So you will have to be master of your own weaponry, too. You must also know vitamin C, know it "cold." You must know the beast and you must know vitamin C. *Knowledge* is your edge, your only edge. Practically everything else favors the cold. Knowledge can come pretty easy to *you*. I'm glad *you* won't have to go through the school of hard knocks I did. Of course there will be more things doctors are going to learn about colds in the future, and I can hardly wait to learn them, but we know enough right now to do ourselves plenty of good. Indeed, that's exactly what we're talking about in this book.

3

What You Should Know
About Vitamin C

"*Doctor, I have never quite understood just
what a 'vitamin' is,*" Grace R., a piano student in her second year
at the local conservatory, said to me one evening during one of our
cold-treatment sessions. "It's not exactly a medicine, is it, because,
after all, you hear that there's a lot of vitamin A in carrots?"

"Well, a vitamin *can* be a medicine, Grace, of course," I
agreed, "but there is a lot more to it than that. I don't know how
much time we should take on it. I don't want to bore you with
too many technicalities. You know, I think *you* could possibly
succeed in spoiling Beethoven's 'Moonlight' Sonata for *me* if you
insisted I study up on all that 'counterpoint' and 'harmony' or
whaterever you call it, in that piece, that *you* have to know in
order to do it justice, but only if you're going to be the one who's
playing it."

"I think it's time I should be able to pin this down more
accurately," Grace persisted, "if I am going to be using considerable amounts of vitamin C—and I'll do *anything* to ward off these
colds. They are such a *waste* of time."

"Very neatly said," I congratulated her. "After years of
putting up with these four and five days at a stretch of feeling
rotten, sneezing, and having to reach for a tissue every 15 seconds,

it all pretty much boils down to just that. A cold is a dreadful waste of your time, at the very least. Who needs it?"

"I take voice, too, Doctor," Grace added. "Most all of us are in the chorus for the experience in ensemble it gives us. And you just can't sing with a cold."

"That's for sure. Well, stop me any time you feel you're getting fed up," I cautioned her, "because the idea of a 'vitamin' is about as easy to describe as it would be to try to explain to somebody on the planet Mars what an elephant is if you can't show him a picture of one."

It would certainly be impossible to try to compress the sizable network of ideas behind such a term as "vitamin" into one short sentence that could possibly satisfy Grace. I was going to have to say, "Well, it's a very large animal, and it's gray, and it has a trunk on this end, and a sort of a tiny pigtail on the other, and its ears flap like huge leaves," and so on and on, until Grace herself would be able to put together a reasonably good picture of the "animal."

WHAT IS A VITAMIN?

"What is a vitamin?" I asked myself aloud. "Well, basically it is a food, that is, a source of nourishment for the body, but it is a very special kind of a food, indeed. While actually only a very tiny amount of each one of these special foods, the vitamins, is needed, that tiny amount is *absolutely* needed. You must have it if you are to stay alive. You can't continue living very long without getting a new supply of this material into your body, nearly every day. In fact, the word 'vitamin' itself was made up of two parts, made up out of two other words, 'vita,' standing for life, and 'amine,' which describes a certain type of chemical. You see . . . ."

"What is a 'chemical'?" Grace interrupted me.

What is a chemical? This girl wants to know what a chemical is, I thought to myself. Whew! That's tougher than defining a vitamin! But what I *said* was:

"Well, everything there is, everything that exists, is a chemical. When you get right down to it, every piece of matter, every substance, is made up out of chemicals."

"Is a piano a chemical?" Grace asked.

"It's a collection of chemicals, certainly," I answered, somewhat lamely.

"Is the human body a chemical?"

"A magnificently complicated collection of great numbers of chemicals, yes. Though at one time the whole bunch were said to have a market value of only about 98¢ put together," I smiled. "Surely inflation has changed all that by now, though. Anyway, I'm glad you brought up the question. For while a chemical is everything there is, we usually mean more by this word 'chemical' than just something sitting there like a lump of lead, doing nothing. When scientists use the word 'chemical,' this word has built into it the further idea that we are going to talk not just about things just sitting there, but about how several things are going to react, the one with the other, about what is going to *happen* when two or more things get together. That's 'chemistry.' "

"Like sodium chloride is plain old table salt?" Grace filled in.

"Yes, even though sodium alone or chlorine alone have not the slightest visible resemblance to the salt in a shaker. Well, now, back to amine, which is the second half of the word 'vit-amine.' Amine is the name for one particular family branch of chemicals. It largely is a description of the building framework (similar to the framework of a house, really) of this particular family of substances. It is sort of a general blueprint or plan of this one family of chemicals, of one family among many other different types of chemical families. A member of the amines has certain characteristics that show it as a member of that particular family of substances, just as, for example, monkeys belong to a particular family of animals. And we use a word like 'amines' for exactly the same reason we use a word like 'monkeys'—to immediately convey to anyone who is familiar with chemistry—or monkeys—all the special characteristics of the particular 'animal' we're talking about without having to go through them all from beginning to end every time we want to refer to this 'animal.' "

"As a matter of fact, Doctor," Grace wanted to know, "don't chemists, the people who study chemicals, actually want to know not just *how* two materials will affect each other when they meet, but also actually what the smaller building blocks, I guess you'd say, are that make up molecules?"

"Well!" I said, trying to sound like Jack Benny when he's being astonished.

"High School Inorganic Chem I," Grace beamed.

"Fine, Miss Roberts." Now I was all encouragement, professor-like. "Will you remind the class what a 'molecule' is, and give an example?"

"A molecule is the smallest division anything can be cut into and still be recognizable as the substance you started with. One single molecule of table salt is still salt, but break this up into an atom of sodium and an atom of chlorine and there's no more salt around."

"And, Miss Roberts, considering we may still have some laggards here today who are more fascinated over our prospects with the egg-shaped ball against Lynn Classical than they are in the structure of the universe, will you also remind us what an 'atom' is?"

"An atom is as small as anything can be split at all, unless you want to talk about 'splitting the atom,' " Grace blushed.

"Is an atom recognizable as something familiar?" I was still acting the professor.

"Yes. Of course it's incredibly tiny, but if you could see it, gold would still be gold. But *almost* everything in the world is not made up of just one type of pure atom—or element—like gold, but is made up of *combinations* of atoms. We call these combinations molecules. Actually there are only about 100 elements, the most basic of all building blocks of matter, but I suppose there are many millions of different *molecules* possible, all of them made up from two or more of the 100 elements."

"Yes, and to steer us back to where we were," (I was a doctor again) "an amine, then, is one of a particular family of molecules having its own characteristic family framework structure, and a 'vit-amine' is a particular one of this amine family which just happens to be a substance essential to human life. *Most* amines, of course, are not *vit*-amines and are not 'essential to human life.' By that phrase we mean that the human body does not possess the power to construct this particular substance for itself, and cannot manufacture it anywhere within the body 'factory,' yet the body must have a supply of this particular material if it is to keep living."

"Then where *is* it manufactured?"

"Well, obviously, it has to be manufactured somewhere outside the human body if it can't be made inside. In nature, that is before humans became smart enough first to learn that such a thing as vitamins existed, and then still smarter, enough to be able to make these substances in a medicine factory—vitamins were originally manufactured within the bodies of certain animals or plants, and we got them by eating the animal or plant, which is still the best way."

Organic Vitamins

"Were vitamins originally obtainable *only* from animals and plants, from something that was *living*?" Grace asked.

"Yes, because the chemical structures of all of the different vitamins, no matter which, are what we call 'organic,' meaning that originally they could be manufactured only in some 'factory' that was itself a living body, be it animal or vegetable. Vitamins cannot originate in nature from minerals (like iron, for example), which are substances that are not alive."

"But now vitamins can be made even in Massachusetts, and out of material that *never* was alive?" Grace smiled a bit triumphantly.

"Some of them, yes, particularly the ones with relatively simple structural frameworks. And vitamin C *is* a rather simply frameworked vitamin. Its molecule is a small one and its blueprint fairly simple."

"Everybody knows that there is a lot of vitamin C in oranges," Grace mused. "How can you call it vitamin C if the orange can manufacture it? I thought you said part of the definition of a vitamin is that it *cannot* be manufactured by a body that needs it? If the orange 'needs' it and yet can manufacture it itself how can you call it 'vitamin' C? That doesn't tally. . . ."

I switched tracks. "A logical mind like that must be a great asset at the keyboard. You have struck right to the heart of the matter. Yes, the word 'vitamin' must include the idea that the particular substance being discussed is both necessary and vital to life in a certain animal (usually the human one). Both necessary and vital to life *in a certain animal*—that's the key phrase—and yet that animal cannot manufacture it for his own use. To a human, this substance vitamin C, for example, *is* properly called a vitamin, but to an orange it is not a vitamin because the orange can make it for itself. To an orange this particular substance has to go by its common chemical name, 'ascorbic acid.' This specific chemical, built with a particular blueprint, is *always* and under any circumstances, and to everybody and to everything (including to both the orange and to humans), this substance is always and forever ascorbic acid, that's always right, but *in addition,* it is also vitamin C as well as ascorbic acid, but *only* to those who both, (1) must have it, and (2) can't make it for themselves (that, of course, is us). This is all merely a convenience, so that we can lump under one general word, 'vitamin,' all of the several necessary-to-life accessory food substances. These very special foods are quite different from each other in many ways, in their structure-frameworks (molecular blueprints), in where they come from, in precisely what it is that they do within the human body, in how much of each is needed, and so forth, but all share the common characteristics that they are absolutely required by the human body and cannot be manufactured by it."

Accessory Foods

"Why did you call the vitamins 'accessory' foods?" Grace asked.

"That's because such a tiny amount of the various vitamins is all that's needed," I explained. "You see, Grace, you don't use vitamins as your main food. Rather they act to help you get the most *good* out of the foods that make up the largest part of what you eat. Vitamins act in your body as what the chemists call 'catalysts.' A good way to understand this is to consider all your regular food—meat, vegetables, breads, whatever—as being the equivalent of your coal or oil supply in the cellar, and the vitamins rather like the match, or spark, it takes to get the fire in the cellar furnace going to start with. No spark—you can't get any fire going. And actually the comparative size of the original match compared to all the shovelfuls, or gallons, or whatever it is, of the fuel your cellar furnace will be burning, is a very good picture of how tiny the amount of the various vitamins you must have to get your body 'furnace' started will be, compared to the amount of ordinary foods you will be eating to 'feed your own fires.' "

Grace looked a bit perplexed. "Then the vitamins can't do you much good unless you have a good bit of food around, too. No use striking a match if you have no wood to burn. I know a girl who's trying to lose 15 pounds, and her diet is only all the water she can drink and her vitamins. Claims she got this diet from a hospital, too. Is she just kidding herself, Doctor?"

"To some degree, yes, Grace," I agreed. "But you must remember that when you're on a diet you *are* eating something. That something is your own stores of fat, and it may well be that you can use your fat a little better if you have your vitamins there to help you. Certainly they'll do no harm. But maybe right here is as good a place as any for me to caution you on one thing. There *is* such a thing as getting too much vitamins. They are *not* completely safe and wonderful things, of which the more of them you get the better off you are, necessarily. They can be very powerful medicines when you get them in the big doses, and this is not always to the good for you. In treating colds, for instance, we use very large doses of vitamin C, and we must take care not to use these large doses any longer than absolutely necessary, nor to continue vitamin C beyond the time it's really needed. This is why it's so important for you to follow the treatment instructions exactly when you're controlling one of your colds with vitamin C."

Grace wanted to know if what we had just been talking about meant that vitamin C did its good work in colds by making it possible for you to get more good out of the food you eat.

Sources of Vitamins and Their Health Value

"I have to admit," I told her, "that our talk did seem to be leading that way, but you see we're talking about two vastly different amounts of vitamin C that we may be using. When we get all our vitamin C from ordinary foods themselves, say one orange a day, rather than by taking pure vitamin C in pill form, then we are getting only a rather small amount of this vitamin. This small amount is plenty to do all of what we would customarily want vitamin C to do for us, on a day in and day out basis. That is, in this case we aren't asking it to help us out especially with the common cold, but only to keep us from getting scurvy (a very unpleasant disease condition we'll discuss later, and which is totally preventable by vitamin C in quite small quantities). Well then, vitamin C from one orange a day is only a small amount. From ten or twenty 250 milligram-size tablets a day of pill vitamin C from a druggist's bottle, that's a very different matter. In this kind of amount we have to think about vitamin C as being a treating medicine and very likely it works in these big doses in an entirely different way from how it works in little doses. I'm quite sure vitamin C does act in a different way in big doses: it exerts its influence *directly* upon some of the body tissues, rather than just influencing how *food* is absorbed and put to use, as it does in little doses. In effect you're comparing one orange against the equivalent of 100 or 150 oranges (vitamin C from pills)."

How Vitamins "Do Their Thing"

"When vitamin C does its trick against colds, it is not merely by allowing you to get more good out of your food. It's doing something entirely different that it can only do in very large doses. While we're on this, have we talked about milligrams and so on, Grace? No? Well, manufactured vitamin C comes in tablets of *differing* strengths, but they all look to be about the same size, very much like an aspirin pill. Whatever part of the pill is not vitamin C is made up by sugar or something equally neutral. So they have to tell us how much power of vitamin C is in a particular tablet, and this is stated to us in milligrams, which is, as you know, part of the scientific measuring system. A milligram is one one-thousandth of a gram. That is, there are a thousand milligrams in a whole gram. A whole gram is itself still pretty small by ordinary everyday standards. It isn't much of a piece of chocolate in one of your back tooth fillings. Milligrams (always abbreviated mg.) and grams are weight measurements with exactly the same kind of continuing and dependable meanings as are weights like pounds and ounces. The reason these scientific weights milligrams and grams are quite small is to make them convenient to be used in discussing *medicines* of various sorts, which medicines are almost always used in ever so much smaller amounts than things like potatoes or beefsteaks are. Indeed it would take about 28,000 milligrams to make one ounce, and some 453,000 milligrams (or 453 whole grams) to add up to a pound of anything."

Grace easily took these figures in.

Vitamin C Dosage Calculation

"So if you have your exact instructions for treating a cold handy, and it is time for you to take 625 mg. (milligrams) of vitamin C, you see that you can do that by using pills of most any available power, just as long as you know what power they are. You can get 625 mg. out of two 250 mg. size pills and half of a third one. Or you could get your 625 mg. out of six 100 mg. size pills and a quarter of another one. It makes no difference. In fact every once in a while one or another agency of the government starts thinking it should allow vitamin C to be sold in only one particular size of pill, say 70 mg. or 100 mg. This happens to be somebody's idea for the month of March, 1971, say, but it's only somebody's *idea* of what the standard 'minimum daily requirement' of vitamin C (M.D.R. for short) should be for a normal adult human being in good health. This whole thing is ridiculous, since there can be no such thing as any absolutely fixed 'requirement' of any vitamin for any one individual, sick *or* well, because individuals differ too much from each other. Humans don't come stamped out that similarly. However, the only point I am really trying to make here is that by the simplest arithmetic, you can make up the particular strengths of doses of vitamin C you need at the time from pills of *any known* strength.

HOW TO GET THE FULL POWER OF VITAMIN C

"And here is another point for you never to forget, Grace," I continued. "It's a most important point. Vitamin C, or using its simple chemical name, ascorbic acid, is a material that is so 'lively,' so ready to go and to start working for you, that if you don't take very excellent care of it, a good bit of it won't be there by the time you get around to using it. This applies whether it's the relatively small amount of vitamin you have the right to expect from a medium-sized orange, or the greater amount of vitamin C you count on getting your full measure's worth from, say, a 250 mg. power tablet. If either the orange or the tablet isn't fairly fresh it is quite likely to shortchange you on your vitamin C. While good amounts of vitamin C are originally present in nearly every fresh fruit, vegetable, or leaf there is, long exposure to air, or heating the food by cooking it will destroy most all of the vitamin C. Actually you have to take better care of your vitamin C pills than you do of your orange, because the orange has a thick skin that keeps out air, light, and even some heat, and you don't ordinarily cook an orange either. So you can see that spinach wouldn't be nearly as dependable as a source of vitamin C. It has no protective shell, and furthermore you cook it.

"It can be disastrous if three or four in a row of your called-for doses of vitamin C while you're treating a cold are supposed to be 625 mg. each, and you combine two and a half of what you think are, and originally *were* 250 mg. tablets of vitamin C, thinking you're getting 625 mg. that way. But if those pills have lost strength down from 250 mg. to say only 100 mg. each now, you have goofed and are going to pay for it. When 625 mg. is needed, then 625 mg. is needed, not 200 or 300. As you have heard before, and will again, Grace, 'halfway' doses of vitamin C in treating a cold are usually completely worthless, they don't give you even 'halfway' results."

"How can you be sure your vitamin C is full strength, Doctor?" Grace asked.

How to Buy Vitamin C

"First, don't try to save money by buying a big bottle of vitamin C. Buy it only in small, that is, one hundred pill or less bottles, which must still be sealed with original paper or plastic seal when you receive them. Keep the still-sealed bottles in a relatively cool (refrigerator not necessary), relatively dry, relatively dark place until you use them. A solid cabinet or drawer, with no glass doors, and not near a radiator will be perfectly satisfactory.

"For treating any one cold use only a bottle you have just personally opened or seen opened, keep it tightly closed between doses, and throw away any pills that are left over at the end of the cold, so that the next time you will again be starting with a freshly opened bottle. Most vitamin C bottles are of brown glass, which keeps out light, and most cap well enough to keep out ·moisture. But still it will be up to *you* to do the sealing of the bottle after every dose. Do it well. Remember that air getting to your vitamin C is probably the worst risk it must face. Properly sufficient vitamin C dosages are absolutely required if your cold is to be successfully treated. How can you possibly be sure a dose *is* sufficient if the vitamin C pills you are taking have lost some undeterminable part of their power through old age or careless handling? You can't."

How Vitamin C Got Its Name

"Why do they call it vitamin *'C,'* and is all vitamin C the same no matter where it came from?" were Grace's next questions.

"It's called 'C' because it was the third in the line, A, B, *C,* the third letter in the alphabet, the third of the main vitamin groups to be widely studied by scientists. Some say the 'C' stands for 'citrus,' for the citrus fruits, oranges, lemons, tangerines, and grapefruit which are such very excellent suppliers of vitamin C."

"Isn't it funny that mothers have been giving their children hot lemonades for colds for heaven knows how long?" my companion mused.

"I know what you mean, Grace, but that's not just the mere coincidence it seems to be. There is some truth rooted in this old wives' tale of hot lemonade being good for colds, just as there has been more than a little truth in lots of other kinds of folklore. There is enough vitamin C in a good strong lemonade to at least ward off, if not finally and completely cure, certain milder cases of colds that happened to get that lemonade at precisely *the* right time. Although most colds didn't noticeable respond to hot lemonade, a few did, enough to start the story going. And those that did respond were responding to vitamin C."

VITAMIN C–THE SAME REGARDLESS OF SOURCE

"Now as to whether vitamin C is the same no matter where it comes from. Yes. It is always the same simple ascorbic acid molecule whether it comes from an orange, from the leaves of a Galapagos Island tea lily, or from anyplace. Man-manufactured vitamin C is identical with that made by nature's factories, and the body accepts it as such.

"Some people think that the ascorbic acid produced by some such exotic plant as rose hips is somehow better than other vitamin C, but that just isn't so. The only fit and final judge of such a matter is the human body, and it has decisively spoken. It *likes* vitamin C, period. While we're on that it's worthwhile to point out that we wouldn't be able to treat colds with vitamin C at all if brilliant scientists hadn't figured out, first, what vitamin C's special blueprint was, and then, armed with that information, gone on to learn how to make it up artificially. Dr. Albert Szent-György won the Nobel prize for his work on this one substance. (Incidentally, this renowned researcher, though he did his vitamin C work some 40 years ago, is still alive and working on new scientific problems, right here in Massachusetts, U.S.A.) Without artificially made ascorbic acid concentrated in pill form we couldn't easily get together the very large amount of vitamin C that is required to control a cold. The big doses of vitamin C needed to treat a cold at its beginning are equivalent to 100 to 150 medium-sized oranges a day. 75 oranges won't do the trick at this stage."

VITAMIN C—THE TESTED REMEDY FOR COLDS

"Does vitamin C do anything besides cure scurvy? Well, *some doctors believe that vitamin C actually will do certain valuable things over and above what everybody already accepts for sure,* that is, scurvy—and these doctors may well be *right,* or some of. them at least may be. But so far as I know, in only one situation has the proper research actually been done. For only one condition has the *full* set of accepted ways of testing a medicine to see if it really can control a disease actually been carried out. That is for vitamin C's power against the common cold. This power has been *proved,* and proved in the only way possible short of 200 years of just sitting and watching.

"Vitamin C can prevent and cure scurvy, and vitamin C can control the common cold. Any and all other claims that vitamin C can help other ailments—alleviate backaches, benefit cancer, block the formation of kidney stones, even cure polio, and a hundred others—must at this time still be classified as only guesswork. I myself am almost certain that vitamin C does have the power to favorably influence some other diseases—these being particularly some among those infections caused by viruses. I personally believe that vitamin C can do other things besides treat scurvy and colds, but I cannot and will not state these as certain facts even though I believe them to be true, because these things have not been *proved* in the customary, required, scientific way. There are some people who actually go so far as to believe that vitamin C can do a great many things that it obviously just can't do at all. These vitamin C 'nuts' have gone *too* far, making almost a religion out of vitamin C in some instances, and this kind of thing has not served the cause of vitamin C well. Such clearly far-fetched attitudes about vitamin C on the part of some of the public are among the reasons why many physicians are reluctant to even consider any new and useful power attributed to vitamin C, even if it be research-proved."

CONNECTION OF UROLOGISTS' FINDINGS TO VITAMIN C

"Doctor," my secretary Miss G. cut in from the doorway, "it's three minutes to nine, as ordered. By the way, I've just opened two more 'urologist letters' that came today."

"A urologist letter, Grace," I explained, "is from a doctor who specializes in kidney and bladder diseases. We've gotten quite a few of them, and they always say the same thing—that one of their patients who is taking a lot of vitamin C regularly doesn't seem to get colds anymore and do I think there's a connection? Of course there's a connection!

"This is a fairly new vitamin C treatment that the kidney doctors have been using recently to keep a person's urine on the acid side, in the hopes that it won't form kidney stones or stones in the bladder. They're about the only sizable group of patients in the country who are regularly taking very large doses of vitamin C, the kind of dose needed for colds, and it's surprising how many of these people have caught on that they don't have colds anymore and then connect it with the vitamin C. It's surprising because there's really nothing to make them connect it with what the doctor is giving them for their kidneys. Of course the *doctors* who have read my report immediately suspect the reason."

"This finishes me for tonight?" Grace started to get up.

"If you pass your test, yes. What is vitamin C? Make it short and better than I did."

"A vitamin is a very special food which you need only an infinitesimal amount of, but you must have that little bit to live, and you have to eat it specially somehow because you can't make it out of your food. Vitamin C is one of these vitamins. It's a medicine used to treat a disease called scurvy, and you say it's been proved to be able to control colds, and it probably can do some other things like acidify a person's urine for certain benefits."

"A-1, Grace," I smiled.

4

How and Why a Cold Behaves the Way It Does

We are indeed lucky to have found a medicine that can acutally *do* something against the whole set of miseries that make up the picture of a common cold, instead of just making a mild, ineffectual stab at one or the other of a cold's many *symptoms. Vitamin C positively does have the power to actually block the development of the cold itself, and to control to a remarkable extent every one of the characteristic distresses that routinely come with colds.*

If you're treating a cold properly with vitamin C you're only very barely aware that you *have* a cold and are progressing through it. Only once in a very great while will maybe one drop of moisture roll down the inside of your nose—once in two days perhaps. And even then this drop is never "itchy." You just *never* have to blow your nose, just dab up one drop after about 48 hours. Nor will you ever reach the stage where you have any thick yellow discharge coming from your nose, which ordinarily happens about the third or fourth day of an untreated cold.

You're very unlikely to have any roughness in your throat at all—if any, it is mighty slight. It is most uncommon when you are on a proper program for taking vitamin C for you to have any trace of hoarseness, either. Your taste and smell remain as good as they customarily are. You just don't have to sneeze or cough. And you don't feel sick. You feel about 99 percent as good as you do when you don't have any cold at all.

In order for you to be able to detect in any strongly convincing way that you really *are* suffering a cold and really are being forced to make your way through one, you have to put yourself to a very strong test indeed to bring it out. About the only thing I've ever been able to find that you can't do just as well when you have a cold and are treating it with vitamin C as you can when you have no cold at all is a really tough mountain climb! This continued dragging of your weight up a vertical elevation, hour after hour against gravity is just about *the* most vigorous physical test you can subject a human body to, a far greater test than practically any other sport or physical work you can think of. And this is the kind of rigorous test it takes to be able to actually demonstrate to yourself that that cold *is* in there somewhere for certain, and is successfully continuing to exert a small—a very small—illness-making influence on you at the moment.

THE CASE OF PETER P.

Peter P., perhaps the most consistently dependable competitor on his college skiing squad, was introduced to me outside the little theatre in North Conway just before the evening show on the night just before the Harvard-Dartmouth slalom scheduled for the next day. At the time he was squiring one "Muffin" B., a college girl from our town, and we were all shuffling along in line to see a movie. I routinely avoid entering this tiny playhouse with its quota of coughs and sneezes anytime the outdoor movie down the street is still functioning.

I once picked up a cold in this closed little box during the showing of another movie. But the outdoor auto theatre was now long closed, and anyway that's what you get for being a movie fan, or rather what you get for not keeping your head about you. After ten years of study and research into colds I had allowed myself to slip a cog, and had not brought along my vitamin C with me in case I were to need it. And I paid the price! I had picked up a cold, though it probably wasn't from the characters in the movie even though they *had* come in a poorly ventilated submarine. And then I had had to go through all the motions of *treating* this cold for over a week, with a lot more vitamin C than the two little tablets it would have taken me to *avoid* it, if only I'd had them with me. But since that lesson learned at such cost, this was one theatre I'd never forget to bring my vitamin C to again, and this time I had it at the ready.

"This is Peter P.," Muffin was saying as we slithered past the popcorn machine. Her boards-on-his-feet-type boyfriend had apparently come completely equipped even to his freshly running nose. The upshot of it all was that I promptly handed over my this-time-remembered plastic pocket cylinder of vitamin C pills to Muffin's drippy-nosed companion, and accepted his invitation to station myself the next day at the bottom of that terrible snow cleft known locally as "Hill-man Highway," to view his per-formance—if any. It really isn't so bad up there in the ravine by April, and besides I was wondering just how our athlete would show, since there's no lift in the ravine and you have to personally drag yourself up to the top of the "Highway" for every slide down.

Well, Peter did seem to labor a bit mounting the 45 degree cliffs of snow to the top of the "Highway." He was passed on the way up every time by other ascending skiers, their skis slung over their shoulders, but his performance on the sticks on the way *down* clinched the day's scoring for the Hanover team. When it was all over I managed to drag myself a few feet up to where Peter was pulling the flags in.

I had worried a little whether the mere 16 hours Peter had had from his first vitamin C dose at the lobby fountain of the movie theatre to the noon gun opening the slalom would be enough, but it had been. "How was it, going up?" I quizzed him.

"Rough, Doc, rough, but except for that I wouldn't have known I had a cold. Great!"

Even though you're still about 99 percent "there" during a cold you're treating with vitamin C, and are able to do just about anything you want with no trouble, still you always know for a fact that you really do have a cold. There's no doubt whatever in your mind that you do have one, you're completely aware of that, but it's not doing anything to you. It gets across to you somehow that that cold *is* going on, you know you have it, but it gets nowhere.

HOW VITAMIN C CONTROLS THE COLD YOU HAVE

All this is to stress that when you have a cold and are controlling it with vitamin C there is no question the cold is really there, even though you're not minding it. It hasn't been absolutely killed outright, and you know and feel this. The cold is being held in check, yes, beautifully restrained by vitamin C, but it's still alive—and still kicking ever so slightly. Your assignment is to see to it that this sleeping, not-quite-dead cold is *kept* that way—forced to mind its own business. If you can keep it roped down long enough it will finally burn itself out and be gone for good without ever having bothered you at all. But to do this you have to realize that you must be able to match your cold step by step.

Relax your vigil once and it's up and running again. When you first try to rope a cold down, that is, when you are beginning to treat it, you have to be pretty rough: you have to use sizable doses of vitamin C and you have to be quite accurate about timing them. Later on when the poor horse is nearly "gone" (the cold almost over) you don't need to hold him roped down quite so hard—your doses are smaller and also further apart.

To be master over a cold then, you must know your "monster," and in this chapter we are going to talk about everything we know about the nature of the beast. We'll discuss all that we now understand about where a cold comes from, and how and why it behaves the way it does.

THE ROLE OF THE VIRUS IN CAUSING A COLD

"They say that colds are caused by viruses. Is that so, Doc, and do I have to know what viruses are?" The questioner was a patient of mine, Mr. Leon A. (When he heard through the "grapevine" that I was doing something new with colds he was quick to show his face after eight years' absence, and he was all ready for a taste of whatever new medical "goodies" might be about to be served up.)

"Well, sir, if I know you—and I probably do—you wouldn't have brought it up if you didn't intend to have it discussed," I opined.

"Well, I am a talker, Doc. You may remember that," Leon agreed.

"I do, Mr. A., I do," I went on. "Yes, colds are caused by viruses. What is your idea of a virus, Mr. A?"

"Well, I know it's something that's mighty small—it's a mighty small germ that can cause a disease."

"Yes, that's exactly so. How small? Could you see it through a jeweler's loupe?" (I knew Leon had been a watchmaker before he retired and decided to get back some of his Social Security.)

"No," Leon said, "I guess not. Much too small for that."

"Could you see a virus through a microscope?" I asked him.

Leon already had a pretty good idea what a microscope was, but in recent years a new and different type of microscope has been developed, called the "electron" microscope. You may not be able to directly "see" a virus through the electron microscope, but you can see them (or many of them, there is some difference in their sizes) in *photographs* made by the electron microscope. This instrument is able to magnify things up to sizes like 33,000 diameters, or even 65,000.

So viruses are very small indeed. Are they alive? Well, possibly, even probably, but we're not absolutely sure about that. Some experts believe that some viruses may have lain motionless in the cellars of the pyramids of Egypt for thousands of years, and yet can still reactivate themselves now. This doesn't necessarily prove they are or aren't alive. What is perhaps more important than whether they themselves are alive or not is the certain fact that they cannot get anywhere or make any progress in multiplying themselves unless and until they can get themselves *into, inside,* a *living* body cell, one of the living small fragments of which all things that are alive, all humans, animals, and plants, are entirely composed.

"Is a virus a single cell?" Leon wanted to know.

"Yes, if it's alive, which I suppose it probably is. A bacterium, or single one of the bacteria, is most certainly a living, single cell," I told him.

The Enigma of the Cold Virus

Do all viruses cause disease? No, in fact it's believed that most of them do not. Only a relative few of all the multiplicity of viruses are able to cause disease in the human body, and while some others can cause illness in animals other than the human, most viruses probably don't cause disease to anything, or at least if so we don't see it that way at this time yet.

"Is it a special virus that causes colds?" Leon was next to ask me.

"To the best present knowledge there are about a hundred different viruses that can be the cause of what we call colds." I said.

"And these other 'bugs' called bacteria don't cause colds then?"

"No, but they can be responsible for the secondary complications that are so likely to follow on a cold," I explained. "Now, *the* most critical thing about a virus for us to remember because it relates directly to our being able to treat a cold successfully, is that the infecting virus must be able to penetrate into the inside of a living cell in the body of the prospective victim. Only within a living, functioning cell can the virus replicate itself."

"What does 'replicate' mean? And I don't know whether I know what 'infect' means either," Leon queried.

"Excuse me," I apologized. "I should have explained that word before I threw it in. I put the cart before the horse. 'Replicate' is a new word meaning that these viruses somehow are, well I guess you'd say, 'manufactured' in huge numbers within the 'rooms' or cells they've invaded. 'Infect,' by the way, is simply a fancy word for a disease bug's invading a victim. The main reason this word 'replicate' was made up to describe the sudden increase in the numbers of viruses inside a living cell is because, as we've mentioned, we're not quite sure that the viruses are alive, so we don't want to use words like 'reproduce' or even 'multiply.'

"Anyway, once inside a cell, within the walls of its little 'room,' viruses seem to be able to take over the facilities of that little room and use them to sort of 'stamp out' great numbers of what you might call carbon copies (or replicas hence the term 'replicate') of themselves. These new viruses once they've completely torn up the whole insides of the 'room,' or cell, in the trick of turning out carbon copies of their own glorious little selves, then they break through the cell wall again, this time in an outward direction. Now the greatly increased numbers of viruses have reached army proportions, and there are enough of them to mount a real attack on other handy cells of the poor victim."

"Does all that happen in a mere cold?" Leon was amazed, "All that drama?"

"It does, yessir," I confirmed. "I was giving you a general description of a sort of model virus infection there, but all that happens in each and every cold."

"Does it also happen in diseases that are caused by other types of germs not by viruses? Does it happen, say, in typhoid fever, where they used to say harmful bacteria had gotten into your water well?"

"No," I told him. "Bacteria do not have to enter living cells to be able to survive, and indeed they don't do so. They can live on the *outside* surface of body cells, or on 'food' they find on the unbroken skin surface, or inside your intestine, in the contents of your bowels."

The Difficulty of Tracing Virus Infection

The fact that viruses ordinarily can survive only if they find living cells to poach on makes them much harder to study, or even to find in the first place, than are bacteria. It was not only because bacteria are usually much larger than viruses—they mostly can be seen through the ordinary type of microscope—that they, bacteria, were discovered years before viruses. Bacteria can be raised (cultured), that is encouraged to grow so we can study their behavior in the process, on such cheap and handy "food" as beef broth or what amounts to chocolate-flavored blood-and-jello. Viruses can't be raised without living tissue for them to work on. Fertilized eggs, that is, the earliest stages of a living chick-to-be, are often used for this purpose, but the growing of viruses is very, very troublesome and relatively expensive, too. And not only are bacteria much easier to study than viruses, they are also customarily a far easier type of nut to crack from the point of view of treating a disease they cause. This is because to kill or "paralyze" *any* germ, you have to "get 'em where they're at." And where *are* they at? Well, bacteria are sitting around loose all ready to gobble up your medicine (which is *their* "poison"). Even if you *could* find a good virus "poison" (which isn't easy) these little fellows have themselves in a great defensive position—safe behind the hard-to-penetrate walls of their living body cells. Yet, that strong defensive position—within the cells—is usually where we would be forced to have to make our attack upon the viruses, if our aim is to seek them out and destroy them. Any medicine designed to attack into this inside-the-cell position must not only be able to dispose of the viruses once it reaches them inside the cell, but would have to be able to have made its way through the walls of the cells without doing them (the cells) too much harm in the process. If a virus medicine were to kill every cell it touches (even though it may kill the viruses inside too) we wouldn't dare to use it. This is because we have no way of making such a medicine confine itself to just those cells containing viruses. The medicine will go everywhere, to all the cells in the vicinity, and do whatever it does to all of them, whether they contain viruses or not. This is too great a price to pay. True, we may be able to kill off a certain number of viruses that happen to be temporarily out in exposed positions where we can get at them more easily.

It isn't too hard to disinfect a drinking glass with enough hot water and soap, nor to clean up a wash bowl pretty well with some strong caustic solution, and precautions like these may very well stop the spread of virus-caused diseases at some times. But in *most* infectious diseases caused by viruses, it is not going to be at all easy for us to get either a disinfecting chemical or, say, some kind of a mechanical block to the passage of a virus successfully introduced somewhere between the person who already has the virus (and the disease) and the other people who don't have it yet.

In most virus diseases the jump of virus from one victim to another is too subtle for us to be able to *see* or even to be able to *time* with any great accuracy, admitting we have no hope of *seeing* the "transmission" (spread) with our own eyes. Not often do we have a situation like rabies (hydrophobia) where we can actually *see* a rabid fox frothing at the mouth sink a fang full of rabies viruses into your ankle. Here, of course, we not only see the transmission of viruses, or at least the act that did it, but we also have it exactly timed. Unfortunately, even with this common chance to view and to date a virus transmission, we probably will have muffed this rare chance to block the spread of a virus by means of some mechanical type of interference with the transfer of the viruses. We should have gotten a muzzle on that fox *before* the bite.

There are also a few other times when we may be able to determine at least approximately *when* it is that a virus passes from person to person, even if we can't see this. But even here we don't know *exactly* when the germ passed and usually we don't even know it approximately until *later,* when the disease has already developed in the new victim and it's too late to do anything about it, at least too late to do anything by way of somehow stopping it *before* it's already made its way safely into the new victim.

But, as we have said, most of the time the spread of a virus from an earlier victim to a later one is usually not visible, nor timeable. However—and finally we're getting a break (it's about time, wouldn't you say?)—we can sometimes—not always, but sometimes—actually see the actual transmission of the very viruses we're most interested in right at this time, those of the common cold. And then we can actually use this sight of a virus transmission to foil the development of a cold, at the extremely low cost of a couple of 625 mg. doses of vitamin C. (This is the "against-a-specific-contact," or "interceptor" dose set. We'll go into it in detail in chapter 7.) These doses must be timed just right—the first one within no more than an hour after the sneeze or cough in our direction. If they are, they will almost without fail keep us from getting the particular cold that might have resulted from that specific sneeze (or, less likely, cough).

IMMUNITY THROUGH HAVING A COLD

Although there may be much variation from one person to another, most individuals, once they have overcome a particular cold, will then enjoy a period of immunity (absolute resistance) to catching a further cold for some time. The commonest duration for this temporary immunity to colds, the length of the protection most people would have, is probably four to six weeks. Temporary it may be, but while it lasts it is a marvelous, nothing less than magical piece of armor—against this one particular type of danger only, of course. The person who is carrying this shield of protection can walk unscathed into the very midst of a regiment of nose-running, sneezing, coughing, eye-watering cold sufferers. He may, if he chooses, rub himself with, sniff up, or even swallow the disease-carrying secretions of the cold-ridden, and will receive no punishment whatever for such daring. The immunity usually extends to protect the bearer of it from colds caused by all of the one hundred different cold viruses, even though the cold which conferred the resistance on him was incited by only a particular single one (or possibly two) of the many cold-causing viruses. Incidentally, you may even be protected, temporarily of course, against some other virus diseases other than colds, too. Of course there has to be some sort of a fly in the ointment, and what it is here is that—at this state of our knowledge at least—we have no known way of determining *when* it is that this remarkable, though short-term, immunity is about to be used up. The best estimation comes from how long it has customarily lasted for you as an individual in your previous colds.

Although it is a very difficult thing to prove in the required scientific manner, there is a very strong impression among doctors that a cold and its following temporary immunity probably also prevents one from catching not only all types of colds themselves, but likely protects you from certain other virus diseases as well for the same period. It is impossible to calculate how many children may have been spared poliomyelitis (infantile paralysis) solely because they happened to have had a cold just before exposure to polio and their short-term immunity-to-colds had extended to protect them from the polio also. (This particular example would of course have been most valuable in the period before the wide use of polio vaccines.)

Why does an immunity established against one cold protect you (at least for a while) against other types of colds, and probably against some other non-cold-type disease viruses as well? Presumably because the original cold stimulates your cells which have been invaded by viruses to produce a protective substance, an automatically manufactured "body medicine," you might call it, which opposes what the viruses are doing inside the cells and finally overcomes them. Once this protecting substance has been produced, it lasts for a while, hence the four to six week duration of immunity. And the protecting substance's action is of a rather general nature, so it works against quite an assortment of viruses, though not all. This protecting, immunity-conferring substance is called "interferon" (pronounced "interfere-un"), because it "interferes" with what the viruses would like to continue doing. Unfortunately interferon is not immediately called forth and produced at the very moment when invading viruses first take over cells. The viruses enjoy a delay of several days of no interference—that is, no interferon as yet—before the protecting substance is manufactured in enough quantity to start fighting the viruses. As your (untreated) cold starts to better itself along about the fourth or fifth day, it is because interferon production has been increasing and has finally reached a useful concentration within the cells.

We have said, then, that there are times when it is, for all practical purposes, impossible for you to catch a cold. Indeed tests have shown that if you take a group of people who do not have colds at the moment and attempt to give them colds as a medical research test you will succeed in giving only about one third of them colds. This is even though you irrigated infected secretions from the running noses of people with active colds into the noses of the ones you were hoping to give colds to. There are probably a number of reasons for this, which we'll touch on again later, but one reason certainly is that some of our cold-free subjects in the test were still enjoying immunity conferred on them by interferon which was produced by a prior cold or possibly some other type of virus infection.

There are scattered individuals—possibly one out of every twenty people, though that may be a little too high an estimate—who never seem to get a cold, or at least do so very infrequently, and this apparent lack of susceptibility (capability of catching a disease) has not been satisfactorily explained so far. Possibly they could have some unknown stimulus in their bodies that tends to give them a nearly perpetual useful level of interferon; of course the real reasons may be entirely unrelated to this possible explanation, which is only a guess.

Children seem to get colds more readily than do adults, but it is hard to tell how much of this apparent extra susceptibility is due to the fact that they are repeatedly thrown together in large numbers in school, and hence have every possible chance to pick up what colds may be in the group overall.

Peak Season for Colds

The peak season of the year for colds is the days and weeks immediately following school opening in the fall. Since the children have just passed through the most cold-free period of the year, a July and August when they can be outdoors (in this hemisphere) and during which they have suffered many fewer chances for contact than at other seasons, hardly a one of them has had a cold for the past two months, and on September 1 practically no youngster scampering up the steps of the elementary school has a scrap of immunity still remaining to him from an earlier cold. So even a single weak cold can wildfire through a school population like the epidemic it really is, and soon be carried back and distributed to the stay-at-home pre-schoolers also, and to parents. Statistics show that Mommy will end up with *twice* as many colds as Daddy. It's her "nurse" job, of course.

In September there is still some useful sun about, and there is also less indoor confinement—with its attendant increase in close person to person contacts—than will be the case by February. So while the *most* colds peak is in early September, the *worst* colds peak is more likely to be in the winter months. It's in January or February that virus respiratory infections seem to hang on and on, and to proceed more often into the secondary bacterial complications of otitis, pneumonia, and so on. September colds less frequently go into these additional bacterial stages. Following the September peak and the depth-of-winter peak there is another high incidence point for colds in late springtime. So that as we follow the year around we observe a total of three peak periods when there tend to be somewhat more colds about than what you might call the usual baseline number for the non-summer nine month period, September through May.

Age Differences in Cold-Sufferers

Just as children seem to get *more* than their fair share of colds, so it seems that those in the much older age groups of 60 plus may get *fewer* than their fair cut. Here again the reason may reside in the number of human to human contacts likely in a particular age group than in any real bodily difference between infant and grandparent. Older people are somewhat less likely to have to venture into the outside world every single day to make their bread or master their ABC's, and are probably more likely to socialize in smaller groups, too. You need eighteen for baseball, but only four for bridge.

Nevertheless, even though the amount of human to human contact that is customary in a particular age group will certainly have a lot to do with how many colds people of that age level are going to get, still it seems to be clear that there really is an inherent (built-in) difference between the young and the old in so far as catching colds goes. Long careful watching of what really happens in life will convince you that, to put it in a rather crudely direct way, viruses prefer young, healthy meat when they can get it. Since they must have living cells to work with, can you blame them for wanting the best, the juiciest?

The common cold seems clearly to be a slightly different disease in youth from what it is in age. Of course the difference is not in the inciting virus, but in the manner in which the victim responds to it, in the way his body handles it. A simple, ordinary, run of the mill cold, with no secondary complication present, will, for example, rarely cause any rise of body temperature in a grownup. Fever in an *adult's* cold almost always means a secondary bacterial complication is present. But the exact same virus, working in the same household at the same time, may cause a baby to run a fever of 102 degrees—often without any complications—and to be seemingly much more acutely sick than is the father of the family.

Aspirin for Colds

Susan L. asked me, "Why do they tell you to 'get plenty of

rest, drink lots of fluids, and take aspirin for the pains and fever of a cold,' if there *is* no fever, Doctor?"

"Because they're selling *aspirin*, Susan, that's why," I laughed. "There isn't much in the way of *pains* either, for that matter. Neither fever nor a headache are prominent parts of a cold ordinarily. But relieving mild pains and reducing fever are aspirin's two strong points, so they ring them in even though they're not the important unpleasantnesses of a cold at all. If a drug maker can't really help a cold with his medicine, why he'll just go ahead and try to kid you into thinking that what his product does help *is* a customary part of a cold, when it's no such thing.

"You remember, though, we mentioned that children, especially small ones, are more likely to run a fever with their colds, though this is usually on the light side. That fever is all right. Don't worry about it. Too many people want to rush to get every fever back down to normal right away. Often that extra heat is part of nature's intentional way of battling an infection. Sure, 105 or 106 may not be too good, though even this usually depends on *why* it's that high and which way it's going, instead of just *how* high it happens to be."

"You don't recommend that aspirin be used at all in a cold? Suppose you had run out of vitamin C?" Susan continued.

"Aspirin is probably the most useful, relatively safe and simple medicine that exists," I said. "We would definitely be worse off if we didn't have it. But, as I've said, its primary values are to reduce fever and to relieve pain of various types, if it isn't too bad a pain, and it seems to have some further quite specific value for various types of arthritis. But as I've also just said, none of these things are characteristic of a cold, usually, not even headache. So I see very little reason to use aspirin. I might use a little of it once in a great while in a child if I *don't* happen to like his temperature too much, but I would never count on aspirin to do anything much for him. If the cold wasn't going well and I was concerned about stopping a *complication*, I'd be using something a lot more effective than aspirin, probably some penicillin.

"But, you see, the average person feels as if he has to do *something* for a cold, and most people don't know *what* to do, so they may take aspirin. *You* do know what to do, Susan, because you're just about to graduate from this particular class in vitamin C yourself.

"Now, what I have been trying to emphasize throughout this course is that I think it would probably be better for you to have to take *no* medicine amounts of vitamin C at all, that is, quite high dosages of it by pill, *if* you can get out of it. And if you do have to take a lot of vitamin C I'd rather see you do that just once in a while rather than practically all the time. Even then you should be sure to take not a bit more than is actually necessary to accomplish what you want to accomplish. Of course, I think a person *should* have the knowledge of what vitamin C can do for colds, since we haven't anything else that's nearly as good as yet, and I think you should use vitamin C and this knowledge on some occasions to treat, and as often as possible to *prevent* your colds. You need not necessarily use vitamin C on *every* occasion to *treat* every cold you ever have. Well, I don't see why I should sit here and bother to be the teacher when I've got a professional teacher right here to do it for me."

THE INCUBATION PERIOD OF A COLD

Gesturing toward Susan, I directed, "*You* conduct a review lecture and session on things like incubation period, infectious period, contagion, inflammation, and such like, and maybe I'll think of something else later. Stay right there because you've already got a softer chair than over here."

Susan took over. "If you want to understand colds, one of the things you have to know about is what is called the 'incubation period' of a cold," she commenced. "Now we all know what an incubator is. It's a sort of warm box that we put an egg into and let it do some developing. What is living inside the egg is growing, and it is making progress, and this whole process is being helped along by the warmth of the box. But the important thing to remember is that what is happening inside that egg, within the incubator, is something that takes not only warmth but a certain amount of *time* to accomplish, and this time must be allowed to pass before we can get our result. If we want the egg to hatch we cannot get out of putting in the necessary time, and the incubator is really nothing but an ideal place for this necessary time to be passed—in a safe place for the egg to be while it incubates, we may say.

"All right now, we understand that. Now let us apply this to the life history of a disease virus, one that is capable of causing the disease we familiarly call the 'common cold.' This virus has been living within the cells of the upper part of the breathing apparatus, or respiratory tract of a certain human, let's call him Mr. A. The virus has given Mr. A. a set of unpleasant discomforts like a runny nose, a cough, and all the rest that we know so well. It's given him a cold. One of the unpleasant things that the virus gave Mr. A. was a tendency to sneeze. All right, he sneezes. And some of the spray from the sneeze is blown into the air right in front of Mr. B., who happens to be standing near our Mr A. Mr. B. breathes in, as he's bound to probably at least 20 times every minute, and some of the spray from Mr. A's sneeze is drawn up into Mr. B's nose and throat, where it comes to rest on the inside surface of these organs. Now this sneeze spray from Mr. A. has in it some of Mr. A's cold-causing viruses, which we know have been developed and made to increase greatly in numbers, and we know this was done within the living cells lining Mr. A's nose and throat. So now we have Mr. A.'s cold viruses sitting on living cells in Mr. *B's* nose and throat. But they're just resting there so far—this is immediately after the sneeze—and furthermore there aren't a great many of these viruses either at this time. Not too many came with the one sneeze. If this was as far as things went, nothing would happen to Mr. B. He wouldn't get a cold.

"If the viruses are to succeed in giving Mr. B. a cold there will have to be a lot more of them, and the few there are now will have to get themselves *inside* of the cells on the surface of Mr. B's respiratory tract, somewhere so that they can make a lot more of themselves. So our viruses have some piece of work cut out for them. First, they must work their way through the walls of some of the nearby cells lining Mr. B's breathing appartus, in this case his nose and his throat. All right, they do this, and it takes some time to do it, although probably not as much as three hours. Perhaps it'll take less than that, but very likely an hour and a half at the least. So now we have a number of the cells on the surface of Mr. B.'s nose and throat with Mr. A's cold viruses inside them.

At the beginning, each Mr. B. cell, if it has any Mr. A. virus at all, probably has only a few viruses, maybe only one. Doctors don't know about that for sure, yet.

"The next step is that the newly-arrived viruses which came from Mr. A., of course, originally—or rather, 'recently' would be a better word, because these viruses or the ones that they developed from may conceivably have been passing through one or another living human for thousands of years in line already—well, the viruses 'take over the management' of the cells, not too differently from how a new manager takes over the direction of a factory. The new virus managers demand that the materials in the cell 'factory' be used to make viruses exactly like themselves. As with any other factory, it takes some time to set up a new assembly line, and then still more time to use it in assembling viruses.

"Now viruses are being made and being stacked against the walls of the cell, readying for delivery, but no delivery is started until a reasonable supply of viruses has been made up. Meanwhile, time is still passing, in fact several days have passed by now since Mr. B. was the receiving target for Mr. A's sneeze, and Mr. B. still feels fine at this point. He has no cold symptoms—yet—and he doesn't feel sick in even the most minor way. He has no idea that the axe is about to fall at any moment. All of a sudden, and pretty much together at the same time, a good many of Mr. B's nose and throat cells that have been turned into virus factories have finally worked up a large enough stock of viruses, and the cell walls are burst open and out rush great numbers of viruses. Right then and there Mr. B. knows he's getting a cold. The incubation period is over. . . ."

"Do they really know that, Doc?" Clifford T., still facing me, interjected in Susan's lecture. "Do they know for an absolute fact that these viruses burst out of the cell like she says and that right then and there is when you feel sick?"

"Well," I explained, "although nobody's *seen* it, the chances are excellent that it's just about that way."

"Well then," Susan continued, "the time between the moment of Mr. A's sneeze, when the viruses were first passed to Mr. B, and the time when they broke back *out* of Mr. B's cells, ready in large numbers to give him the characteristic illness, that is the incubation period. It's the time from the first receiving of a disease-causing organism to the appearance of the recognizable, fully developed sickness. This length of time is not the same for different diseases. What is it for colds?"

"Two to five days," Leon parroted out of his past attendance at numerous of our gatherings.

"Yes," Susan moved briskly forward. "And this means *what* about those movies where a fellow is caught and chilled in a deserted castle by a sudden rainstorm at midnight and then he wakes up the very next morning with a sneezing cold?"

"It means that he *didn't* get the cold from being chilled by that rainstorm, even though the story said he did," Clifford volunteered.

"Correct," Susan pronounced. "When your cold begins it means that almost certainly you picked it up at least 48 hours before that time, but definitely not as much as a week before, either. If you're afraid you might have caught a cold at a particular time, say a certain sneeze you couldn't avoid, and if you get through five full days and the cold has not blossomed out by then, you missed it. What is the *most* likely length for an incubation period, Doctor Régnier?" Susan threw the ball back to me. "I don't believe you told us."

"For a cold I'd say two and a half, three or three and a half days are more likely than a short 48 hours or the longer four or five day stretch," I reported.

Chill as a Cold Factor

"Doctor, is there or is there not anything to this chill business in getting a cold?" Leon put in his five cents worth of question.

"It's interesting that you asked that, Leon," I observed, "because many people aren't really sure what the real truth is on that point, and even some doctors will haggle about it every so often. First of all, I think we ought to point out that the reason this thing is called a 'cold' is not alone because people sometimes noticed that they happened to have been chilled some short time before the cold appeared but also because when you have a cold your temperature mechanism may be shot and you may feel cold sometimes, even though a thermometer will prove that your temperature is normal. This isn't too common in a cold, actually. Lots of times you won't notice this particular cold feeling at all."

"You can't get the cold without the germ, anyway, Doc," Clifford contributed. "You gotta have the germ there."

"Amen is all I can say to that, Clifford," I conceded. "People can stay in terribly cold places for months at a time, and they may be chilled again and again, but if they don't freeze to death in the process—or even if they do—they still won't get a cold if there are no viruses around. This has been shown many times. When Admiral Byrd had his expedition at Little America there would be quite a few colds at first, but after about six weeks they would taper off and there would be no more. Everybody there would have worked through any cold viruses that the members of the group happened to have brought in with them at the beginning from the good old warm United States. There was nobody left without enough immunity to be able to successfully resist the viruses because everybody had already met these viruses and, after suffering colds, had beaten the viruses. With no place to land, these original viruses—the ones brought in at the beginning of the expedition—simply folded up and disappeared. Having no living cells of the proper type—the type they like, those of the human upper respiratory tract—except upper respiratory cells that had become immune to them, they had to call it quits."

Susceptibility to Colds

"How about the guys who had the colds in the first place, who maybe had them when they got there?" Clifford queried. "Why couldn't *they* get them a second time around, if say, six weeks had passed and they'd lost the resistance by then, like the kids in school?"

"Mrs. T., will you answer that question for us?"

"Well, first, you're dealing with adults and they just don't seem to have as much susceptibility to colds as children," Mrs. T. said. "Then I'd say it would be because in a group of that size—I believe they had something like no more than 30 to 40 men on those South Polar trips—they probably would have *all* gotten the cold before the first ones had yet lost their interferon. Or maybe interferon really does last a little longer against the particular bug that caused it to be formed in the first place. Could that be possible, Doctor?"

"I don't know whether it could be possible, Mrs. T., but I do think you've given a brilliant answer," I complimented her. "Well, to continue, here we have these fellows down there, they've all worked their way through the cold viruses they originally brought in with them, and they get no more colds even though some of them get badly chilled from time to time. But let a couple of new replacements come in from *Big* America, and every one of the first comers will soon come down again with colds. Since the original men could have stayed there forever by themselves and gotten no more colds, no matter how chilled they might get, we know that the new arrivals must have introduced some fresh viruses into the society. And this same thing happens every time a new group reports in from home. Surprisingly, it also happens even if not a single one of the new men seems to have an active cold. This last point positively proves that there must be such a thing as carrying a cold virus and not being affected by it yourself, at least at that time. In this situation one at least of these new men who just came in must have been 'silently' carrying a still-infectious cold virus."

"Still, getting yourself very much chilled has nothing to do with getting a cold, right, Doc? It's all bugs." Clifford was happy.

"No, not quite, Clifford," I was not pleased to have to deflate him. "I'll get on with that in a moment. Give me just a moment more before we have to leave Antarctica.

"In the early days exploring ships were sometimes frozen in and had to stay in the Arctic for as much as four years at a stretch. (That is, of course, the *northern* cold place, while *Ant*arctica is the southern one.) No humans were helicoptered in in those days, and for all that time, four cold *years,* the crew, no matter what other problems they may have had, very soon after the beginning had no more colds. There was nobody to bring them any new ones, and the old ones were gone. If a strain (a particular family) of cold viruses can't find susceptible living cells to live on, and find them almost continuously, that particular bunch will usually 'die out,' if you want to say it that way. Those viruses from the Pharaohs' tombs *may* be able to clam up and survive twenty centuries—or that may be all the bunk—but we're pretty sure cold viruses can't. We can't really say for how many tens of thousands of years the human species and maybe even the Missing Link right before him in evolution may have been suffering from colds, because colds leave no certain traces on the old archeological skeletons we dig up, but probably colds have been with us for a very long time. And for all of that time, however long it was, the viruses usually had to be holing up in some living human being. It's possible they may have been able to go inactive for *short* periods from time to time, and *temporarily* survive without any living cell to poach on. Indeed, modern scientists have found that a cold virus, *if* it's frozen and dried, may remain able to come alive and cause a cold after several months of being *outside* any living human cell. But always remember, even if a virus may be able to survive for short periods outside a cell, it can never replicate itself into battle numbers again without cells to seize and use as factories. All right then, as a usual thing we're going to find our common cold viruses holding forth in some living human cell. Notice I said 'human.' No animal the first humans had with them was good enough to do the trick."

Catching Colds from Animals

"You can't catch a cold from your dog or cat, because they don't get them," I went on. "Cats occasionally seem to sneeze but this is not a cold; it is probably an irritation akin to a human's sneezing when breathing pepper. Indeed, very few animals at all are susceptible to colds. This is one of the difficulties in research on colds; there are few suitable animals that could be used for tests with colds and cold treatments, tests whose results could reasonably be applied to humans. Certain types of monkeys catch colds, but they are very expensive animals to use in research. Other, cheaper ones like ferrets may have some type of susceptibility in some organs, but they don't make a good comparative test that could safely give us information useful to man."

"Animals make their own vitamin C. Could there be any connection?" Leon posed at this point.

Temperature Factors

I answered, "The fact that very few animals get colds may have nothing whatever to do with the fact that almost all animals have present in their bodies at all times some ascorbic acid, which, as you say, they can make themselves. Possibly a better reason for animals not catching colds might be their higher body temperatures. Dogs normally run about 102 degrees, for example. Or there may *be* a relationship, or a partial relationship between this animal freedom-from-colds and their having always ready within them the same vitamin C that has such striking power against colds in the human. We can't say yet.

"Recently a report written by doctors, research men, appeared in a medical journal, and a highly respected one at that, and in it these fellows said that they had conclusively proved that chilling has nothing whatever to do with getting a cold. They're wrong. What they didn't understand well enough are some of the exact details of how a cold is actually passed from one victim to another. We've talked about this process of virus transmission more than once, of course, and we have learned that the overall physical and medical condition of the prospective next victim, *does* count in whether or not he is going to catch the cold that is being offered him, for example, the amount of any resistance he may still have on tap from his last cold.

"When a person has been chilled to any considerable degree for any fairly extended period—if you want it more precise than that, let's say he's been shivering in 35 degree cold in a 40 mile per hour wind on the summit of Mount Washington for about an hour—a situation like that will drop the temperature of our hero's nasal mucous membrane as much as ten degrees and then the walls of the surface cells are definitely less resistant to the assaults of viruses trying to invade the cells than is the case when the human body has not been so chilled. As soon as our cold friend is thoroughly warmed up again, these cells will soon return to their normal level of resistance to virus passage. But if he runs into viruses *while he's still chilled,* he's more likely to take in a sizable dose of them than if he weren't chilled. You confirm this association between what a person has been doing and his likelihood of getting a cold, not by setting up a small scale experiment in a laboratory, a set-up that unavoidably must have many artificial features in it, but by *observing* what actually happens out there in the so much bigger laboratory of life itself, life as it's really lived by the human kind.

"In the world we may see and judge for ourselves *thousands* of instances, not just four or five isolated individuals boxed into a room somewhere for only a short period of time. If a doctor wants to really know about a disease like a cold, which while it's not fatal, is really a very complex, tricky deal, he's going to have to get up off his duff, shed his white coat and get out there with the people, the real people. And while we're on this, I regret that we have to go back and slightly modify what our little teacher was telling us some time back about the fellow soaked to the skin and spending the night in the abandoned castle. When he got that cold the very next morning, yes, surely he hadn't caught it in the cold rain only those eight hours before, he most certainly had picked up the germs at least 48 hours previously, probably more, but that chilling he got *could* have made the cell walls easier for the viruses that were already being developed inside to break *out* and thus appear to rapidly give him the cold. When a chill weakens cell walls it makes it easier for a virus to go either way, both in *and* out. Indeed, in the castle story the chill *can* be said to have shortened the incubation period a little, if you like."

"So it does matter if you get chilled, after all," Clifford recorded in his mental fact box.

"Well, it *may*," I said. "It *may* matter *if* you happen to meet up with viruses while you're in your temporarily weakened condition, or if you have some already. But I ought to repeat that for it to matter you have to have been somewhat cold for some length of *time*. Cell resistance to virus passage probably doesn't drop until your chilling has lasted a while. That reminds me of an interesting little point I perhaps ought to put in at this place. When a person is on a reducing diet, if he's really sticking to it and actually losing weight pretty steadily, he can definitely pick up more colds more readily than he would if he weren't losing weight. What could be the reason for that, Clifford?"

"That's easy, Doc," my truck-driving friend answered. "If he's reducing he isn't eating much and undoubtedly his 'motor's' slowed down, just like mine would if there was poor gas or too little gas in my gas tank, and when your motor slows down you're gonna run cooler."

"I knew you could answer that, Clifford," I approved. "So that in effect your body, while reducing, is relatively chilled all the time and supposedly the resistance of the cell walls to viruses will suffer accordingly."

Body Temperature During Dieting

"Is the body temperature of a person on a diet really lower than usual?" Mrs. T. asked. "Can you see that with a thermometer?"

"Sometimes you can," I answered, "by perhaps a half a degree. But even if you can't see it, it makes no difference. Even if the temperature is normal, the overall heat production of a human body on a strict diet is far lower than usual. Isn't that right, Cliff?"

"Sure, it's right. That's what the thermostat is for in a car or truck," he explained. "It'll hold the same temperature through a lot of different heats, and won't let the gauge rise unless the heat you've got way outstrips the ability of the cooling system to adjust for it."

"Surely one of the greatest skills one could possess during the 20th century is a wide comprehension of the internal combusion engine and its workings," I observed by way of appreciation for Clifford's help. "But marvelous as Clifford's truck's thermostat is, his own personal thermostat is far more wonderful. It will hold the proper 98.6 body temperature, or the slight variations in it that are normal through the 24 hours of the day, to a superb degree of accuracy. But while the body can hold its temperature steady at normal, its remarkable capacities *are* somewhat limited and it can't make something out of nothing. It can't make as much overall heat as usual out of less food than usual, and on a diet you do catch colds somewhat more easily. Well, I've taken the rostrum away from our teacher for quite a spell. Susan . . . ."

THE INFECTIOUS PERIOD OF A COLD

"Our next subject," she began, "is an important one indeed if we really are interested in catching as few colds as possible. We must recognize that not everyone who has a cold necessarily has the capacity to give it to us, at least not at all times. Just as we, the persons who may receive the cold, are not always able to catch it, for some such reason as our still having some immunity, so also the person who has a cold may not always be able to *give* it to us, or at least he's not very likely to. A person with a cold is not equally infectious during the whole length of that cold. What does 'infectious' mean?"

"It means 'able to infect,' or in this case, able to give you a cold," the senior member of the group correctly responded.

"Yes," Susan continued. "A person with a cold is most able to pass it to others when his cold is in its early stages. That would be about the first two days of the cold, when a person is liable to be sneezing. Of course, as we have learned before, sneezing is not the only way in which a cold may be transmitted, though it's probably the most dramatic way. Let's each one of us give an example of how a cold may be transmitted. I'll start with drinking out of somebody else's glass."

"Kissing somebody."

"From a cough."

"Going to a dentist who doesn't bother to sterilize all those drills he sticks in your mouth."

"All right, we're glad to know about that," Susan went on. "These then, are just some of the ways you may pick up a cold. Is a cough a very likely way to catch a cold?"

"No, it isn't," Leon quickly said. "Even though I gave that as my example, I know you're not as likely to pick up a cold from somebody coughing as you are from somebody sneezing. That is because a cough is usually one of the later-developing symptoms of a cold. It usually comes later than sneezing, and by this time the cold sufferer is not as likely to be infectious as he was earlier. Also, of course, a cough is usually less of an explosion than is a sneeze, so it doesn't spray all about, and also, I think, most people are more likely to cover a cough with their hand than they are to stifle a sneeze, which often comes on very suddenly."

Catching a Cold from a Carrier

"Could I put in something here?" I petitioned Susan. "Leon is certainly right about a sneeze being sudden and an explosion. I can vouch for that personally. I remember once long ago when I had had my ribs bashed up playing football and then happened to pick up a cold. The sore in my chest from the bruising had been coming along pretty well in the last few days, when suddenly one afternoon I had to let out with a violent sneeze from my cold. That sneeze put so much sudden pressure and tear onto my rib cage that it put my ribs back two weeks of healing and hurt like crazy. I'm not trying to tell you that vitamin C would have prevented me getting bashed up, of course, but it sure could have kept me from ever sneezing that sneeze that did the real damage."

Susan continued: "I'd like to say a little more about this interesting question of catching a cold from a person who doesn't seem to have one at all, at least not in any way that you can see as yet. The doctor was just telling us in reference to the South Polar expeditions that the answer to this question seems to be yes you can, sometimes, from a carrier. Well, ordinary people right here in ordinary situations, people who don't have to be classified as carriers, just ordinary people who are about to come down with a cold themselves, *they* also can give you a cold *before* they even can be seen to have one themselves, though usually they'll be breaking out with it visibly in a couple more hours, isn't that right, Doctor?"

"Yes," I agreed. "And I'd like to say a little more about this, too. Not only has *experience* taught us that it is possible for us to pick up and catch an as-yet invisible cold, at least during the several hours just before it will break out and *become* visible, as Susan says, but you might be interested to know that the researchers have also proved this scientifically by producing colds in subjects of an experiment who have been given nose wash samples from apparently cold-free but really contagious persons."

"*I* also would like to say a little more if everybody else is going to," Clifford T. snorted. "Maybe this 'silent' fellow who gave you the cold you couldn't see *is* going to come down with it in a couple of hours himself, but a fine lot of good *that'll* do if you've meanwhile gone your own way, and don't even know that you've run that risk. Of course, it would be okay if it was your wife or somebody you'd know about. You could take vitamin C and catch it."

"That's one of the toughest things, what you've brought up right there," I observed. "What do you do if somebody in your own house shows up with a cold? It makes a tough decision for you. You know you could take a single 400 mg. of vitamin C, and hike yourself out of there and you wouldn't get that cold, But most of the time you don't care to leave home just for that. What else could you do?"

Susan said, "Be especially careful about dishes, towels, and so on, and stay as far away as you can from the person with the cold. After all, if you're the mother and your husband has the cold, you don't want it, not only for your own sake, but you don't want the children to get it."

"Let the one with the cold move onto the sun porch," Leon offered.

"Grin and bear it," Clifford T. said.

"Of course," Susan went on, "you have the option of taking vitamin C but taking it only until such time as you judge the one with the cold is no longer infectious. That's one of the ways you could approach this kind of situation. You needn't necessarily just sit there and await developments, to see if you get the cold, and then have to commit yourself to a full 12 day treatment course of the vitamin. You can take the bet that you'll be safe if you take vitamin C only until the one with the cold seems to be getting over it."

Then the talk seemed to reach a stopgap.

"Does anybody want to say any more about this?" I looked about. "All right, I guess I'll have to say it myself. If the one with the cold happens to elect to go on a good vitamin C treatment *himself* there's not going to *be* much of a problem within about 18 to 24 hours, is there?"

"Oh, you're right, you're right," Susan took back the initiative. "In an *untreated* cold the victim *is* liable to be infectious for perhaps 48 hours, for two days plus, let's say, after the symptoms begin. But on a good vitamin C treatment the sufferer is likely to be pretty well toned down within only 24 hours, so if you don't want to catch his cold you might need to be especially careful or to take vitamin C yourself only for that long. It might be worth going to the sunporch for that long a time. Does everybody understand, then, that under ordinary circumstances, with no vitamin C treatment being used, a person who has a cold is

probably infectious only for a period stretching from about two
'hours *before* his symptoms appear for the first time, to about two
to two and a half days after that?"

"I think we should say he's not *very* likely to be infectious in
those two hours before his own cold breaks out, really," Mrs. T.
put in. "The hours *after* the symptoms come are much more
dangerous to other people than what you might call those 'silent'
hours."

Susan accepted this modification and was about to go on
when Clifford turned to me and said: "Doc, I'm a little confused.
First, we seemed to have decided that you aren't going to catch a
cold unless you happen to run up against somebody who has one,
and even then you can't catch it from him except for *part* of the
time he has it, the most active part of the cold, the sneezing time
usually, and now we seem to be taking a lot of this stuff back and
saying you *can* latch onto a cold at other times, when there's
nothing to be seen of one around at all."

"Well, you see, Clifford," I answered, "first, we had to try to
get ourselves a clear understanding of the usual, much more
common ways that you are *most* likely to pick up a cold for
yourself. Then, when we had a pretty good grasp on this what you
might call a standard way of catching a cold, we could then go on
and consider some of the more far-out facts of life about how you
can get one.

"Let me tie this together for you a little bit," I went on.
"Certainly the common cold virus is one very slippery customer,
or rather a basketful of them. Actually it seems there may be at
least as many as three different situations where it is possible for
you to pick up a cold when you haven't even been near anyone
who has one, at least one that you can see and therefore try to
avoid. Maybe there are more than three such situations. The *first* is
from a carrier as shown in Admiral Byrd's camp. The *second* is in
the several hours just before a cold that *will* appear hasn't quite
appeared yet. And the *third* place, I'm beginning to think, is where
you can sort of catch a cold from *yourself*. By that I mean I'm
becoming surer and surer that sometimes at least, it *is* possible for
you to carry a virus around on you for quite a time without it
doing anything to you, and then having it break out on you into a

real cold if you slip up and let yourself get tired, chilled, or your nose and throat excessively dried out—or possibly lose your last remaining trace of interferon. I *think* I'm right about this. I don't think that it's just that you picked up some new virus, freshly arrived, and fell victim to that. I think that you finally succumbed to the one that has been sitting there all along, just waiting for you to get careless *and* succumb."

CONTAGIOUSNESS, INFECTION, AND INFLAMMATION

Susan continued: "There are a couple of other words we should understand too, while we're dealing with this end of the subject. The doctor used the word 'contagious' a few minutes ago.

" 'Contagious' means a disease can jump from one person to another quite easily, and likes to do just that. There's more of the idea of the *easy* transmittal of a disease in that word than there is in the word 'infectious.' 'Infectious' means a germ-caused disease too, yes, but it doesn't necessarily imply how readily it will jump from one person to another. In a sense all infections are contagious, but we restrict the word 'contagious' to those that really get around fast.

"Now who will define 'inflammation'? How does it apply to the common cold?"

" 'Inflammation' comes from the same word as 'flame,' " Leon offered. "When a body tissue was swollen, reddened, and hot, it was only natural to think of it as sort of 'burning.' "

"Yes," Susan agreed. "Most all the symptoms that we know all too well in a cold are the result of some part of the upper respiratory tract being swollen, heated, and reddened by the blood supply's having brought in extra materials to the sick part in an attempt to rid the sick part of whatever's annoying it. This is called inflammation. Let's take turns giving examples of it in the common cold. I'll start with sneezing: here the inside of the nose has swollen and the body reacts as if it were trying to get rid of the 'extra' tissue by exploding it out of the nose."

"Hoarseness," Mrs. T. gave in her turn, "means that the vocal cords have swollen due to inflammation and cannot vibrate as cleanly as before, so the sound of the voice is muddled."

"A cough," Clifford said, "is an attempt to clear the swollen breathing tubes."

"A sore throat," Leon explained, "hurts because the nerves in the throat are unduly stretched by the swelling of the throat tissues."

"Runny nose," Mrs T. was on her second time around. "Extra fluids brought by the blood to the inflamed place 'overflow' and leak out your nostrils."

"The discharge tends to become thick and yellow," Clifford was up for his repeat, "when the extra inflammatory materials brought by the blood have more solids in them and less watery fluid. The yellow, which is the same thing as you'd call pus, is made up mostly of white-type cells that circulate in the blood. This thick discharge is a later stage than the earlier watery type."

"Trouble with breathing," Leon brought in. "The breathing passages are swollen shut so that it is hard to draw air in through them."

"Wait a minute!" Clifford T. ordered, "The inflammation of *what* part spoils your taste when vou have a cold? Your *tongue* isn't swollen, that *I've* noticed."

"You principally get your taste not from your tongue, Mr. T.," Susan explained to him, "but from your nose, which *is* swollen, of course. There are taste buds on the tongue, yes, but the receptors in the nose are more important to the sense of taste."

Smoking Factor

"Does smoking give you more colds?" Clifford posed. "I gave it up two years ago now, but I've always wondered about this."

I picked up the ball. "Well, what would you think if you knew that smoking tends to dry your throat, as we all know it does?"

"I'd think a dry suface would probably let the bugs in, if it's supposed to be wet," Clifford said.

"And you'd think right. A mucous membrane lining, which is what the upper respiratory tract is lined with, is properly supposed to be lightly moist. Drier spots are easier-to-penetrate spots. Some statistics claim that smokers aren't any worse off with colds than people who don't smoke. I don't believe it for a second. Anyway, I'm not going to smoke even if they can show me statistics that prove it's good for me."

WHY COLDS VARY IN SERIOUSNESS

"Colds do vary one from another in their seriousness, Doctor," Mrs. T. presented. "I suppose there'd be a lot of reasons for this?"

"Many. How many and which particular viruses you got in the initial 'gift.' What degree of vigor those viruses may have developed while they were in the last victim just before you. What your own general health level and your interferon standing might be at the moment. The condition of your upper respiratory mucous membrane, as determined by such things as how much smoking you've been doing, or whether you happen to be chilled at the very time the viruses reach you.

"Also, so little a thing as whether or not you happened to have very recently drunk a quart of orange juice at just the right time. I remember reading a book—it was the truth, not a novel, and it was a best-seller—where the heroine had been looking forward to a very special date for weeks, and when the time came she very reluctantly had to call up the gentleman friend and tell him to cancel the reservations at the Brown Derby, because she was coming down with a cold and felt rotten. Instead of going out for a lovely evening she found herself squeezing a big pitcher of orange juice and crawling into bed to suffer out her cold. Within three hours she felt so vastly better that she got up and made it to the filet mignon after all. To this day, she sees no connection between the orange juice and her sudden recovery; she didn't put it together, but of course *we* do.

"A million things can relate to how bad any particular cold will turn out to be, Mrs. T. Of course, let's not forget the factor of what any steady day in and day out *preventive* dose of vitamin C you take can do to lighten a cold, if it didn't block it out completely."

"You know what I've noticed, Doc?" her husband spoke. "Colds don't always start the same either. Sometimes it's the runny nose first, leading to the sore throat later. Other times it's the sore throat first. Sometimes you get a lot of laryngitis, other times practically none. It depends on where the varmints hit, right?"

"Exactly so, Clifford," I agreed.

"Referring to this girl who drank the orange juice and then popped into bed, does rest *do* anything for you, really?" Susan wanted to know.

"What it does is to keep you out of circulation. *That's* good," Clifford piped up.

"I like your comment, Clifford," I agreed. "You have pointed out something that is not nearly as much appreciated as it should be. Since colds are spread by droplet infection, if only people with them would take themselves completely out of circulation, they would be making a great contribution to the rest of us, both those of us at home with them and those who must go to work with the victim. But instead of that, somehow by bearing a cold you're supposed to get all kinds of credit for manfully just bulling your way through it, and the fellow who has the cold views himself as a self-sacrificing good sport for going to work instead of retreating to bed, and he expects to collect a certain admiration from all his associates. Instead of being congratulated for his courage, this creature *should* be kicked in the tail for subjecting everybody else in the office to the chance of catching his cold. He is actually nothing but a thoughtless menace, and it is time he was labelled as just that. It is also time for his employer to be willing to encourage him to stay home the next time. It would save the boss money in the long run if his workers didn't trade each other every cold they've got."

Bed Confinement Does the Victim
of a Cold Some Good

"Furthermore," I went along, "although you might not think so at first, going to bed does do the *victim* some slight good, too. Bed rest may not have any real effect on the basic cold, but it's good because this confinement cuts down your chances of taking on *bacteria* that could attack your virus-damaged, sensitive mucous membrane and lead to possible complications. Prevent complications and you'll suffer the shortest, least annoying cold possible under the circumstances.

"Of course all this discussion refers to a cold that has to be allowed to run an unmodified course, as nature would have it. If you can get to a cold rapidly with vitamin C, the whole thing becomes a horse of a different color as soon as you have gotten yourself through the first 12 to 15 hours it takes to snap the cold into line. But to get back to you, Susan, I know why you asked that question about bed rest just that way. You're thinking of when they start to tell you—since they have nothing better to tell you—to 'get plenty of rest and drink lots of *fluids.*' Well, if that fluid happens to be lemon juice and it comes by the *gallon,* yes."

"Same thing would go for 'feed a cold and starve a fever,' right, Doc?" Clifford smiled, pleased with himself. "As long as the food was oranges by the barrelful, how about that?"

"My one grandson never seems to get rid of a cold, or hardly ever," Leon interjected. "I don't understand it, if you say a cold is supposed to last perhaps four to six days and that should be it."

Colds Allergies

"He probably has an *allergy,*" I told him. "It's pretty hard to tell some allergies from colds at times because both have runny noses as a prominent symptom. But plain ordinary colds just don't continue indefinitely. If no secondary bacterial complication like, say, an ear involvement develops, a cold on its own should be pretty much over, ordinarily, in, as you say, in no more than five to seven days."

"That what *his* doctor said, too," Leon confirmed. "You fellows stick together."

"Tell you something," I let him in on some professional secrets, "*if* we seem to stick together on a diagnosis, on what we think a disease is, at that time at least we're probably *right.* If you go to ten different doctors and get ten different answers you'd better start being wary. Somebody's wrong, probably all ten of us."

"Do kids with allergies also get more colds, or worse colds?" Leon pushed along in the same direction.

"I don't believe I can tell you that for sure," I admitted. "Some doctors think they do. But I can think of why in some instances it could very well be true that they might *miss* getting a cold they'd otherwise get, just by virture of *having* an active allergy."

"How?" Leon asked.

"You tell me, sir. Does this youngster's nose run a lot?" I questioned.

"Yes, I guess you'd say it did." Leon was thoughtful. "Oh, I see what you're getting at. If his nose is running it may wash out cold viruses before they can penetrate."

"How do you know that cells affected by allergy aren't *more* likely to accept viruses than usual?" Clifford T. broke in.

"I don't, Clifford," I conceded, "so maybe we better get off this discussion. However, there's perhaps one useful little gem to be mined here that we ought to mention. If you've been sneezed at, you should purposely blow your nose a couple of times in the next five minutes. It could blow off some viruses.

"And now to my little checklist here. You people have been so thorough about it here today that I find only a couple of tiny items that you *haven't* dredged up during the hour. We've certainly touched most of the bases this time. One question I'm usually asked is—'Do colds occur all over the world, and what effect does the climate have on them?' Well, they do occur in the warmest tropical climates as well as in the Arctic, and in the middle, temperate zones between, of course, where most of us are right now, and in all these places they behave *pretty* much the same once you've got one. Colds do tend to be a bit shorter and less severe in the warmest places near the equator, that's true. After all, this is perpetual summer. And there seem to be fewer colds in these warm places, too. This may not be entirely the bright sun there. It could be the greater average intake of naturally-occurring vitamin C that people in sunny climes routinely enjoy, automatically. If there's a very long growing season in a place like Hawaii, it's hardly possible for you to *avoid* getting more fresh fruits and vegetables than an Eskimo can possibly draw from *his* environment.

"One thing that is quite clear: the *complications* of the common cold—the bacterial ear, lung, and throat infections that are so much worse than the unadorned cold itself—are ever so much more a problem in the colder climates, the further toward the poles you go. The Eskimos have a simply terrible record of otitis and mastoid diseases. It's even worse now in modern times than it was in earlier years. Before the Eskimos met up with civilization they lived in individual igloos isolated from any other family, and they ate their seal and polar bear meat *raw* because there wasn't enough fuel (seal oil) available to waste any on cooking, only on a little flickering light. *Uncooked* polar bear meat contains vitamin C; there's practically no other source of the vitamin available in the far north other than raw meat. And huddling together in frozen wooden shack villages hasn't improved their record on the common cold either.

"Those peoples headquartered near the equator have a strikingly different and better experience with the complications of colds. Complications are relatively few and far between in these torrid regions. For example, here mastoid trouble is very infrequent.

Sun Bathing

"Does it do you any good to bathe yourself in sun once you have a cold? Not a bit. Once those viruses have gotten that far along inside you, burning yourself to a crisp will do not one thing so don't bother. The sun is worthwhile only *before* you get a cold, it will probably help you avoid one—if you get enough of it continuously—but sunlight 's vor th not a whit in overcoming one you already have.

"One fellow once asked me, 'Has a cold ever killed anyone?' Well, it may have, someplace back there in the dim past. Certain tribes of Indians who had had no experience before with some of the white man's diseases often died from virus diseases that very rarely killed those of European racial background, mild diseases like measles, for example. It's conceivable that colds somewhere in their long history may have struck a prime target, and decimated a population that hadn't met up with them yet."

THE IMPORTANT LESSONS OF THIS CHAPTER

What are the principal, and most importantly, *useful* things we have learned from our lengthy examination of the usual behavior of this monster of ours, the common cold? Here they are:

(1) The basic cause of a cold is a particular set of germs called "viruses."

(2) These viruses usually can survive only if they have continuing access to susceptible, living human body tissue, which means that to be able to live they must frequently jump from one human "home" where they have worn out their welcome to another new, more welcoming one, a person who has no immunity to them, at least at this time.

(3) During the attempted jump from one person to another we may be able to intercept the viruses and physically stop them, as by wearing a mask over the nose and mouth, or by carefully washing a common drinking utensil. Or that at the time of the attempted jump we may be able to *avoid* the virus even if we can't stop them, as by turning away from a sneeze.

(4) And now a *most valuable* piece of information: the viruses of a cold on their first arrival at the upper respiratory tract of the prospective new victim—you—will for a short while be forced to be in a relatively unguarded position (before they can penetrate the cells) and that we may have a golden opportunity to catch them at this point (by taking a special "interceptor" dose of vitamin C; see chapter 7).

(5) If all else fails and the viruses probably did successfully cut through our every defense and did successfully invade us after all, we still have a breathing space of a minimum of at least 48 hours and a maximum of five days before they're going to make us actively sick, a knowledge we may sometimes want to put to good use by immediately finishing up something that would be difficult once a cold had developed, such as sending our weekly "letter" of voice tape to that boy on duty in Germany.

(6) And, of course, a magnificently *useful* thing that we have learned, or at least again been reminded of, is that we have the power to force even a developed cold into submission with enough vitamin C, if it be our choice to do so. (For treatment see chapter 5.)

(7) Once we have conquered a cold, whether it be with the help of vitamin C or not, we have earned ourselves a ticket of freedom from further colds for a stretch of weeks, very probably.

5

Exactly How to Beat Your Cold Using Vitamin C

At last we're about to be served the meat course. Right here and now is where we're going to find out *exactly* how to go about really *using* vitamin C to master *your* cold. Here are the A-B-C to Z instructions finally. To ensure that you'd get good results with them, and not be disappointed with the outcome of your first vitamin C battle with the common cold, all of the previous explanations really *were* necessary.

For one thing, now you have the background to be able to understand and to handle any odd little departures from the standard, expected, what you might call "normal" behavior of a cold being treated with vitamin C. You'll know that such and such a funny symptom is not important, even though you can't call me on the phone person-to-person to ask about every little twinge in your left funnybone as the friends in my original research groups could. Anyway, by far the most of these little "funnies" my patient-friends wondered about had nothing to do with either the cold or with the vitamin C treatment it was getting. Such little items were usually traceable to a mother-in-law, the boss, or the next income tax bite.

But there *are* a few little things—odd, though usually tiny, headaches, and muscle twinges located in unaccustomed places which really are due to the combination of the cold and its vitamin C method of treatment. It's important for you to recognize that these can occur and not to worry about them. Okay, so I can't be on the other end of the phone for you, though I dearly wish I could be, because I like to talk with people. Anyway, everything that I could call upon to answer your questions is somewhere in this book already, and if you've read it you can get the same answer I'd give you over the wire. Let's go on with a brief, overall look at what we're going to be doing as we treat a cold with vitamin C.

THE CASE OF MARGARET G.

Margaret G., was chief of check-out girls in our local supermarket. Wrapping an arm protectively around "Sapphire," the cat, Margaret settled into a purple overstuffed cube of chair and requested of me, "Give me the barest outline on this vitamin C business, will you? You can flesh it out later."

"Okay Margaret, that's a reasonable request, a quick outline," I conceded. "If you have a cold and you want to treat it with vitamin C, and if it isn't more than about 24 hours old so far, what you're going to be doing is this: You're going to be taking vitamin C for a total of about 10 to 12 days, and you're going to be taking it every three hours, day and night around the clock, except that you don't have to take a middle-of-the-night dose if you don't happen to wake up. You may have your full eight hours of sleep unbroken. *If* you wake up you'll take a dose, but you won't wake up especially for that. After about three days on the beginning size dose, you'll cut down on the size of your vitamin C doses, and if you get away with that lesser dose size, you'll cut *it* down still further after about another three days. Then perhaps in another two days after that you'll cut it down again, and then again until you're finally taking very little. In other words you're cutting down on the amount of vitamin C that you use as the cold fades out. What you're really doing all along is using only enough vitamin C to hold the cold in check until it dies out of its own accord. If you've gotten away with all this according to schedule you can then stop the vitamin C completely, as I say it'll be about 10 to 12 days after you began. By this time the cold will be thoroughly burned out. That's about the size of it, in the barest bones."

"What can I expect from my cold if I keep up this treatment as directed?" Margaret wanted to know.

"I'm sorry to say that you can expect to not get out of a single day of work. You will report to that office daily as usual, and continue with your ordering and bookkeeping, because you just won't feel poorly enough for even one moment to feel that you can excuse yourself from *anything*. If any of the girls goof off it'll even be back on your feet and out to the register for you. That's the kind of shape you'll be in, right through the whole cold."

"I don't want to stand there blowing my nose," Margaret protested.

"Give yourself 12, or maybe 15 hours at the beginning where you're just starting vitamin C, and there'll be no more nose blowing or anything else."

EXACT DIRECTIONS FOR BEGINNING TO TREAT A COLD WITH VITAMIN C

(If you with the cold have already taken your first two doses of vitamin C according to the permission granted in the Introduction, then please bear along through these paragraphs with those of us who are just about to start *our* treatment, until we catch up with you, ready for the third dose of the treatment six hours after beginning.)

The following conditions must be met if treatment is to be successful:

1. You must have had the cold for no more than 24 hours.
2. You must have *fresh* vitamin C available.
3. You must understand milligram measurement of dosages.
4. You must not have eaten a large amount (more than 1/2 pint) of yogurt or buttermilk in the last eight hours.
5. You must be pretty sure this *is* a cold, the kind of thing *you* have when you have a cold.
6. You must have no specific disease of your digestive tract (such as a stomach ulcer).

And now for some details on these cautions.

> *ONE: You must have had the cold for no more*
> *than 24 hours—that is, you must have had*
> *the visible symptoms for no longer than*
> *that*

Let's return again to one of my research group:

Charles M., age 17, a bright high school senior asked me, "Suppose I've had the cold *more* than 24 hours? I must have *some* chance to control it with vitamin C, or *some* people must have anyway. Surely the chance to control a cold doesn't suddenly bang shut right at 24 hours. The human body doesn't work that way."

I minded not at all being instructed in the intricacies of behavior of the human animal by a stripling so young I could easily have delivered him into the world myself, and the reason I didn't mind was because he was both bright *and* right. "I suppose you want it in exact percentage points, don't you, Charles?" I answered. "Okay, just as a practical guide, here it is."

CHANCES OF SUCCESSFUL CONTROL OF A COLD BY VITAMIN C

1. Treatment begun within the first 24 hours of a cold:
   95 per cent chance of success, with good results appearing within 12-15 hours.
2. Treatment begun only at 24 to 48 hours after cold appears (the second day):
   About 35 per cent chance of success only, and this only after a long delay, possibly as much as another day and a half (36 hours).
3. Treatment begun only into the third day of the cold:
   Success rate nearly invisible, less than 1 per cent, don't bother!

"I'm sure, Charles," I told him, "that I can count on you to get started within 24 hours, usually, or to make the judgment that since you're too late you'll pass on treatment this time."

"How much of an effort *should* one make if he can't get to treating a cold until the *second* day—how far should he go before concluding he's missed the chance?" Charles persisted. "You say there's a 35 per cent chance there. Suppose I've been out backpacking and didn't have any vitamin C with me, but I'm back where I can get some now on this second day of my cold?"

"I'd say you're a scamp, that's what I'd say!" I told him. "A several days' supply of vitamin C would weigh probably all of one ounce. You couldn't get that into your pack somewhere? Do you like sleeping out on the ground with a stuffed-up nose?"

"All right, up to that point I goofed," Charles conceded, "but now here I am back and smart again, and ready to do what you tell me on this second day of the cold."

I counselled: "I customarily tell people I don't consider it worthwhile for them to try to control a cold with vitamin C if you get about it only on the second day. Let's look at it this way: after all you've already suffered through one day of the cold, and even if you're going to be in the lucky 35 per cent, you won't be getting good results for as much as 30 hours *after* you do begin vitamin C treatment—this *second*-day beginning—so there's at least another day that you'll be having cold discomforts in no way softened from a completely untreated cold. I guess *that's* the question you were asking, Charles. Even if you're going to get good results, it'll take over a full day for them to begin. By that time you'll already have enjoyed a full-fledged type of cold for better than two days. It's just not worth the bother to try to solve a cold that's been present for over a day, for over 24 hours. Just admit you missed it, and do better next time."

"But if I want to try?" Charles pushed me.

"Well, start the vitamin C schedule just as if it were a first-day beginning, but if you're not making a striking improvement within 24 hours you are almost certainly done for as far as this cold goes. Get off vitamin C and forget it this time. One thing I am very insistent upon: I never let a first-time user of vitamin C to treat a cold begin on anything but a very early, first-day cold. They'd be too likely to get no good out of the treatment if the cold is over 24 hours old, and would be disappointed and immediately dismiss vitamin C as another flop, another failure in an unbroken list of failures at treating colds."

TWO: You must have fresh *vitamin C available*

Vitamin C is a substance that rapidly loses its power if exposed to air or heat. Since the size of the dose is critical to the success of the treatment—dose by every single dose—the *only* way we can be absolutely sure of getting enough vitamin C at a particular dose, the only way we can be sure of getting the required amount for that dose, whatever the required amount is at that time, is to have really *fresh* vitamin C whose power can be counted upon to be what it's supposed to be, or the alternative would be to take a vast overdose of questionably powered (old) vitamin C. That latter choice is a poor one, since we don't want to take more of the stuff than is absolutely necessary. Too much of it is not all to the good, we must never lose sight of that.

A Nurse's Cold Experience

"Doctor Régnier, your treatment failed me this time," Mrs. Mary T., a recovery room nurse favorite of mine sniffed at me outside the operating suite of the hospital one day, her nose slightly W. C. Field-ish looking and a tissue at the ready in her hand. "Last time it worked fine, but this time no go."

"Where did you get the vitamin C you used this time?" I asked.

"I didn't have enough of my own left at home, so I pieced it out right from the hospital pharmacy downstairs," Mary said pertly.

"Mary," I lightly scolded her, "the hospital buys everything in one thousand tablet bottles at least, opens them and leaves them open for months at a time. That works for most drugs but not for vitamin C. No wonder it didn't work. What about the ones you had at home? Where did *they* come from?"

"Oh, that was a great value, Doctor," Mary gleamed at the memory of it. A 250 count bottle for only $1.69."

"Then you had some vitamin C left over from your last cold," I calculated. "Which was how long ago, about?"

"Oh, it was last spring. I haven't had a cold since then," Mary proudly reported.

"So *that* part of your vitamin C, too, Mary, was out of date. If you want to get the results *you must have full-strength vitamin C* that you've personally supervised from the moment the originally sealed bottle was first opened. Now, you buy bottles of no more than 100 tablets each," I ordered her, "and you immediately throw away any part of one of these bottles that's left over at the end of any one cold. You won't lose much, and you'll have the assurance that you'll *have* to start treating your next cold with full-strength vitamin C."

> *THREE: You must understand milligram measurement of dosages*

If you don't feel perfectly clear on this, re-read that part of Chapter 3 of this book before you go on.

> *FOUR: You must not have eaten a large amount of yogurt or buttermilk in the last eight hours*

Many people like these foods made from milk (and harmless bacterial cultures) and feel that they do a lot of good, particularly in keeping one's digestive tract "regular." One way in which they do keep things moving along nicely in the gastrointestinal tract is by forming curds, and these masses of digesting milk-food stimulate the intestine to contract and push things along in the proper direction. But the curds also have the shape and consistency to "absorb" or hold onto some of the other things that you have eaten, and in this manner some of the vitamin C you have swallowed to control your cold is detained for a while, and kept from reaching your blood stream as soon as it should. The net effect is that the level of vitamin C in your blood is lower than it would be if no yogurt had been present in the intestine, and indeed the vitamin C is too low to keep controlling your cold. So the best thing to do is to avoid eating yogurt or buttermilk entirely while you are trying to *treat* a cold you already have. If you have a considerable amount of these foods somewhere in your digestive system at the time your cold breaks out and shows itself, it will be difficult to tell exactly how much effect in lowering the power of your vitamin C tablets will result. But the longer it's been since you ate these curd-forming milk products the more likely they're far enough along not to interfere too much with your being able to absorb vitamin C in your intestine and get it to your blood stream where it can be carried to the tissues of the cold-sick, virus-infected nose and throat. Of course, don't eat any more yogurt once a cold has shown itself, and you'll probably do pretty well if you simply *double* the size of the first three doses of vitamin C you take in treatment. Yes, make your first doses 1250 mg. each. Then return to the recommended schedule, at 625 mg. dose sizes.

FIVE: You must be pretty sure this is a cold, the
kind of thing you have when you have a cold

This is, of course, because vitamin C is by no means a cure for everything in the world, and if you are using it in a manner designed to control a cold, then you better have a cold. Not that it will do you much harm if you don't have a cold, but it most likely won't do you much good either.

SIX: You must have no specific disease of your
digestive tract (such as a stomach ulcer)

This much vitamin C may irritate a gastrointestinal system which has disease-caused raw surfaces within it, and before using the large doses of vitamin C needed to control a cold, a trial test should be conducted using a much lower dose of vitamin C.

ACTUAL TREATMENT OF A DEVELOPED COLD WITH VITAMIN C

The First Three Days of Treatment

As the treatment schedule starts, if you are ordinarily a very heavy meat eater, cut back on the amount of fibered (muscle) meat (and fish) that you eat and hold your consumption of this at a modest level for the length of the treatment. Particularly limit yourself on *ground* fibered meats such as the ever popular hamburger. These meat restrictions have nothing whatever to do with the effectiveness of vitamin C's action against a cold, but you will probably be more comfortable if your diet has been modified in this way. We'll go into the reasons for this later in this chapter. No other change in your diet is necessary, and you may eat as much *non-fibered* protein such as eggs and cheese as you care to.

How to start treatment

To start the treatment take 750 mg. of vitamin C with as

much water (or other drink) as you need for the swallowing. Three hours later—to within an accuracy of no more than five to ten minutes either way—take 625 mg. as your second dose. Continue every three hours thereafter with another 625 mg. until bedtime is approaching. If bedtime happens to fit just about right on your every-three-hour schedule of doses, you take the expected 625 mg. again, *if* you feel that you'll surely be awake again anyway within three or four hours from then. *Don't* set the alarm clock specially. Take another 625 mg. at the proper three hour interval in the middle of the night, and still another one three hours after that, exactly as if it were daytime and you hadn't gone to bed at all. This is, of course, *if* you are awake at the times anyway. It won't hurt if it happens to work out to a four hour interval between doses during these few *nighttime* hours. But see to it that the larger daytime part of your schedule is well kept to the every-three-hour dosage plan.

At Bedtime

Now, on the other hand, if at bedtime you're pretty sure you'll sleep through until morning, then make the last bedtime dose 750 mg. instead of 625, and make the first dose on your wakeup eight hours or so later another immediate 750. These two increased 750 mg. size doses will successfully bridge the missing dose in the middle of the night for you. Three hours into the next morning you go back to the 625 mg. level doses all through the day, at three hour intervals, just as you did the first day.

Now what do you do if the bedtime dose *doesn't* just happen to fit pretty well tailored to your three hour schedule of doses? You will have to make an adjustment so that what you take right at bedtime will pretty closely continue to keep up the vitamin C in your blood to the right level. This is what it is that you've been doing by taking three hour doses of vitamin C continuously—keeping up the level of the ascorbic acid in your blood to the necessary strength to bring you the results you want against colds.

So if three hours *hasn't* passed since the last (625 mg.) dose you took, you must adjust the bedtime one down somewhat, accordingly. Let's say you are the wakeful type who'll surely be awake from time to time during the night, and thus comfortably be able to keep on a three hour schedule all through. In that case, if only an hour has passed since your last daytime dose, then cut your at-bedtime dose two-thirds, that is, take *about* 210 mg. (Anything that averages out between 200 and 225 would be good, of course; make an "error" upward in dose strength rather than downward if you can't hit it on the nose for accuracy.)

If two hours have passed since the last before-bedtime dose, then we piece out by taking about 420 mg. as the at-bedtime dose. We won't specialize it further than these three choices of dose size at bedtime (approximately 200, approximately 400, and 625). Nor will we bother with half-hours, etc. Remember we've been talking about the wakeful type here. What we have just said presumes that in the dark hours after bedtime you will again be awake to take 625 mg. at three hour intervals, or you could take 210 at hour intervals or 420 at two hour intervals, those would work just as well. The only reason we don't do it that way all around the clock, that is, use one or two hour intervals between doses, is that we want to make it as easy as possible for ourselves, and doses at three hour intervals are as easy as it is possible *to get good results from,* providing you are using ordinary tablet vitamin C.

Doses at four hour or greater intervals—when used on any continuing basis—simply do not work well enough, no matter how large such four-hour-or-longer doses may be. (This is one reason why vitamin C has failed to do anything for colds for some people in the past; they took it with too much time between individual doses.) The underlying reason why you must take vitamin C every three hours—or more frequently—is that your very efficient kidneys strain all the "extra" vitamin C out of your blood, leaving only the "standard" amount of ascorbic acid in your blood, and they take about three hours to do so. It is the job of the kidneys to regulate the amounts of all sorts of things in the blood, and a pair of healthy kidneys (or a lone one, for that matter) will hold all the many chemicals in the blood stream at or very close to their proper levels. Of course when you're trying to treat a cold you have a special reason for wanting a higher-than-normal level of vitamin C in the blood stream, and the only way to get it is for you to more than out-match the kidneys' splendid abilities to keep vitamin C—and everything else—down to the normal level.

All right, if you're the wakeful type then, you pass through the night by taking some vitamin C from time to time, as the interval from the last dose you took calls for. You will keep up a good high blood level of vitamin C in this way. Now let us go back to the dead-to-the-world sleeper type who won't wake up all night. You remember that if his schedule fits just right, if at bedtime it's close to exactly three hours since his last dose, he would be taking 750 mg. to go to sleep on. Well, if his schedule doesn't fit right either, he also will make an appropriate adjustment to his scheduled bedtime 750 mg., depending on how long it's been since *his* last dose. But in any event, this deep sleeper can't cut it much, because he is expecting to pass the night without awaking to replenish the vitamin C level in his blood. So if his last dose was two hours ago, he better take 625 anyway to face up to the long night and if his last dose was only an hour ago he still better take in at least 500 mg.

What we have said so far, then, carries both of our nighttime types—the heavy sleeper and the light-and-interrupted one— successfully into their second day of treatment, which will continue according to the same schedule and at the same dose size as did the opening day. In fact, this beginning plan is to continue unchanged until three full days, 72 hours from the beginning of treatment, have passed. Only then are we going to cut the doses down some.

Recapitulation of first stage

To recapitulate this first stage of our treatment, we begin it at the very beginning with an extra big (750 mg.) dose, and then, in effect, settle down to 625 mg. size doses every three hours around the clock for a three day stretch, modifying this dose size a little only to accommodate our established sleeping habits, in the evening and on arising.

Results of the First Three Days of Treatment

What results do you have a right to expect in this first three days of vitamin C treatment of your cold? Well, in something between 12 and 18 hours of the beginning of treatment, just where depending largely on how many hours the cold had been allowed to run before you started vitamin C at all, and usually nearer the 12th hour than the 18th, all the symptoms of a cold that you had been having will start getting better, and no new ones will appear. Very probably by the time 24 full hours of treatment have been accomplished, you'll hardly know you have a cold.

But it is true that during these first three days of vitamin C treatment, there will be times when you will get the idea, though not very strongly, that the cold is really just below the surface, it's still there, and it's struggling to break out again, if it can. These times of increased awareness that the cold isn't very far away—*if* you have them—tend to be toward the end of each one of the three hour periods of treatment. Just before it's time for the next dose is when you may feel that you surely do just about need it again. In that case, it is indeed a pleasure to look forward for the few remaining minutes till the next dose, to your soon being able to take that vitamin C, because you know what it will do for you—slap the cold down again for another three hours.

The Second Three Days of Treatment

Three days of vitamin C treatment have pulled the cold very well into line, and now you can cut down the dose size. You will go to 400-420 mg. doses during the daytime, still keeping up the three hour interval period. For the night, if you are the sleep-right-through type, you again modify the bedtime and on-arising doses away from the routine 400-420 just as you did the first three days, adjusting them to roughly 2/3 of what they had been during the first three days, that is, you take 500 mg. for these last and first-next-day times.

If you get by on this fourth day of treatment with this lower dose level of vitamin C, with no reappearance of cold symptoms, you will stay at this same 400-420 mg. level for two more days, which will bring you to the 7th, 8th, and 9th days of treatment.

The 7th, 8th, and 9th Days of Treatment

For these you will cut the vitamin C dose still further, to 200-250 mg. size, and still at three hour intervals. Remember you will still be having slightly larger doses than these at bedtime and on arising if you are the sleep-right-through type, approximately 300 mg.

The Final Days of Treatment

When you've finished up eight or nine completed days of treatment, you'll slack off still further with the medicine. How do you decide whether you should make this next drop in vitamin C dosage after *two* days, or after three days of being at the 250 mg.-each-three-hours level? Well, by how you're doing. If you just don't seem to have any cold anymore, no sign of it, no trace, you can make the cut in two days; if you're distantly aware still that the cold is still smoldering quietly underneath there somewhere, then wait for three days. In either event, you can now, on this 9th or 10th day of treatment, for the first time safely go to a dose interval a little longer than three hours if you want to. You can take 250 mg. every four hours instead of every three hours for say just a single day, and then go on taking the 250 mg. size pill at only six hour intervals for perhaps the final day of treatment. Or if you don't mind frequent dosages even when they're no longer necessary, you could still stick to three hour intervals, taking 150 mg. each time instead of 250 at four hour intervals, and then for the final day you could use 100 mg. every three hours instead of 200 every six hours. In these last days when the cold is close to burned out, the vitamin C dose is no longer so very critical as it was at the beginning, in either size or in timing.

You have completed the treatment, and it has lasted overall some 10 or 11 days. It has enabled you to pass entirely through a cold without suffering any curtailment whatever in your usual day to day activities. And in the process you have earned exactly the same temporary immunity that will protect you for a while at least against the next cold as you would have gained had you struggled through the cold in the ordinary fashion, untreated by vitamin C. That's the story, and almost everyone who's tried it, and tried it *correctly*—following the instructions implicitly—has found it a very pleasant kind of story indeed.

Now I think it would probably be quite helpful to review some of the things about this method of treatment for colds; things that have been brought up by my patient-friends while they were learning the techniques of the treatment for their first time. To make it snappy, we'll just identify them, and let them present their situations or pose their questions, and we'll then get about answering it with the least possible ado so that it'll be most worthwhile for you who are reading and hearing about these things for *your* first time, too.

#1
WHAT HAPPENS IF YOU DO NOT CARRY YOUR TREATMENT OUT PRECISELY AND ACCORDING TO INSTRUCTIONS?

Tom R., age 35, medical lab technician. "I was doing very well the first two days, but on the third one I began to get my runny nose back, and my throat roughened up a little. I suspect that could have been because I got a little sloppy and missed one dose and was late on a couple of others, because when I went back to being more careful again things straightened out—but it took half a day for me to get back to where I had been before I got careless with the dosages. It took that long for my nose to dry up well again, and the throat condition to disappear."

Answer: Tom, laboratory chemical tests on samples of your blood, the very same tests that you yourself have often done in the lab for patients, will show that the level of ascorbic acid (vitamin C) in your blood plasma (the liquid part of the blood) will fall back pretty much to its normal level, which is not very much, within about three hours after you've taken even a quite large dose of vitamin C (by mouth, that is). Thus these laboratory proofs nicely *explain* what we already have learned to be true in the actual treatment, that is, that regular doses of vitamin C have to be taken at three hour or *shorter* intervals, not at intervals greater than three hours between doses, no matter how big the doses may be. If you slip up on even one dose, expecially near the beginning of the treatment, it is going to take you extra time to recover your position, as you, Tom, have just pointed out to us.

#2
WHY DON'T WE USE A SUSTAINED RELEASE CAPSULE OF ASCORBIC ACID TO TREAT A COLD?

Doctor Demos K., anesthesiologist (and a darn good one).

"Ed, why don't you use a sustained release capsule of vitamin C instead of those every three hour doses, especially at night?"

Answer: It is obvious to any doctor that a long-acting type of vitamin C dosage for the common cold might be able to simplify the treatment schedule considerably. Such a sustained release capsule would presumably need to be taken only three or four times a day, that is, possibly every six or possibly only every eight hours. But no such capsule was yet available during the major portion of the time I was doing my studies on treating colds with vitamin C. So as yet there hasn't been time enough for anyone to work out a treatment schedule using long-acting capsules that could safely be recommended to the general public. Indeed, even given time, it might prove difficult to work out a plan using sustained release capsules, a plan that would give consistent enough results, because these capsules, though they are designed to dissolve rather slowly, do not necessarily dissolve at the same rate in everybody's stomach. The blood level of vitamin C resulting from using them might not constantly remain high enough to do the trick against colds, for *some* of the persons following a particular recommended dosage schedule. On the other hand a dosage schedule using ordinary white-tablet vitamin C and using it at three hour intervals is quite a bit more likely to give a very high proportion of the people following it good results.

As a matter of fact, as it was one of the largest pharmaceutical firms in the country, a prominent manufacturer of vitamin preparations had to specially make up tens of thousands of test capsules for me, according to my own design, so that I could even start conducting my research work and have it match up to established scientific standards for such tests. The vitamin C in these special pills was ordinary vitamin C, the same *you* can buy at your nearest drugstore, and it couldn't be something that wouldn't be available to the public. If I *could* work out a successful treatment for colds using a certain medicine, what good would it be for you if *you* couldn't get the same medicine?

Very recently one drug manufacturer *has* brought out a sustained release (long-acting) form of vitamin C which does keep up a pretty good blood level for up to eight hours for many people. I'm sure these capsules can control a cold satisfactorily, but it will again take considerable time to work out, again in actual patient tests, what timing and dosage schedule will deliver the best results, *consistently,* in the treatment of colds. And it's possible, as we've already said, that any one schedule using this form of the vitamin might not work well for *everyone.* This is because, as we have said over and over again, the dose of vitamin C has to be just so—enough and timed quite accurately—if we hope to keep up the continuously high vitamin C level in the blood stream that is needed to keep a cold controlled within bounds.

I have already satisfied myself that these capsules (they have 500 mg. of vitamin C in each, packed in a way to release it gradually over a six to eight hour period) can immediately be applied to the *nighttime* portion at least of our treatment schedule. But you see, it took me nearly ten years of experiments to gradually perfect the overall, round-the-clock treatment schedule that I'm recommending to you in this book. By now I'm quite sure that *that* works well. Proving out a good working, around-the-clock schedule for the long-acting, sustained release capsules as a treatment for colds wouldn't take anywhere near another ten years, but I'm not ready to make my recommendations on it to you as yet, and meanwhile I don't think you should be deprived of the chance to use vitamin C for your colds any longer. You really just don't need the sustained release capsule at all if you will up that last at-bedtime dosage and the first at-wakeup-in-the-morning one, as we have discussed, or, of course, if you're the awake-all-night type. But if you wish to use long-acting capsules for the nighttime, take three of them (1500 mg.) as your bedtime dose, and you'll need no ordinary (tablet, fast-acting) vitamin C at that particular time then. This, of course, would be in the *first* three day stage of treating a cold, where you are using 625 mg. as your regular every three hour dose during the day. Your first dose the next morning should again be the standard 625 mg. of ordinary, tablet vitamin C. For the three nights of the *second* three day stage of your treatment, that is, days 4-5-6, where your daytime every three hour dose is at the 400-420-450 mg. level, the bedtime sustained release capsule dose should be two capsules, and for the 7th, 8th and 9th days of treatment, *one* long-acting capsule at bedtime.

Actually the sustained release capsule would do us more good if we could safely use it in the daytime rather than to cover the nighttime hours, because we already have a good enough way to spare ourselves getting up at night especially to take a dose. *If* we can get the long-acting capsule worked out for a successful daytime use, it would cut down the number of dosages we have to remember by at least a half. I'm all for that.

If you want to play around yourself with the long-acting capsule for possible day use, I'd suggest you don't try it until you've had the experience of treating at least perhaps five or six of your own colds with the ordinary tablet, so that you have established a clear idea of just how much vitamin C at its best and most dependable will do for you, that is, the "standard treatment." With that as a background you'll be able to know whether you as an individual are doing as well as can be expected when you're using your long-acting capsules, or whether you should make further changes in the regime you've been trying.

3
WHAT TO DO ABOUT HEARTBURN WHILE YOU'RE TAKING LARGE DOSES OF VITAMIN C

Alan S., 19, engineering sophomore. "Doc, I found after a couple of days that I'd get heartburn for a while after each dose of vitamin C. It isn't very bad, but what does it mean?"

Answer: First of all, the heartburn means nothing as to the way the vitamin C is holding your cold in check, as you probably noticed. The cold is being well-controlled.. Second, one *good* thing heartburn means to me is it proves you have been keeping up your doses, both as to size and timing. Otherwise you wouldn't get the heartburn—and incidentally, only about one quarter of the people I've treated have ever had heartburn under these circumstances, as an accompaniment of vitamin C treatment.

What caused the heartburn? Well, the vitamin C caused it, undoubtedly, and it can sometimes cause it even if you did faithfully follow my suggestion to cut down on your eating of muscle-type meats while you're on vitamin C for your cold. To reduce your chances of having heartburn was one of the reasons I advised you to hold back a little on steaks, hamburger, and the like. If you didn't do that, do it now. That alone may get rid of the heartburn. If it doesn't, and the heartburn really annoys you, you can take a teaspoonful of baking soda in water from time to time. Or it is sometimes helpful to take smaller doses of vitamin C at more frequent intervals. If you're on 450 mg. every three hours at the time you get the heartburn, change it to 150 every hour. This amounts to the same thing but often gets rid of the heartburn.

Even if you do nothing—continue on ten hamburgers a day and take no baking soda and don't retime your schedule to hourly intervals—the heartburn will go away as you advance to smaller and smaller vitamin C doses, as your treatment plan calls for, of course.

4
WHAT ABOUT GAS IN THE STOMACH WHEN YOU'RE TAKING LARGE DOSES OF VITAMIN C?

Miss Grace B., 27, bank secretary. "Doctor, it seems to me that I have considerable gas in my stomach. Is that connected with my taking vitamin C?"

Answer: Yes. Some people on large doses of vitamin C will notice that they have this, though most of them won't. I'd like to say right at the beginning that those few who do notice this gas consider having it to be far better than having to endure an untreated cold, once they have seen what vitamin C can do to spare them the usual cold symptoms. As to the gas, there are two explanations for this extra gas in the gastrointestinal tract while you're on vitamin C. One reason isn't important at all, but the other could be. The unimportant reason is unimportant because it will most certainly stop as soon as you quit taking vitamin C. It is this: large doses of vitamin C tend to slow the "motility" or natural constrictions and relaxations in the intestinal tract that help to move your digesting food along it. Any such slowing of intestinal action, whatever the reason, always results in some extra gas.

Let us all understand that a certain amount of gas in the gastrointestinal ("g-i") tract is a *normal* situation, it's not wrong. How much gas is there depends a great deal on the *type* of food you've been eating lately. Some foods form gas directly by being irritating to some people's intestines. An example would be cabbage, which doesn't necessarily annoy everyone, remember. Some foods promote extra gas in a more indirect fashion—they do it by especially favoring the growth of certain of the bacteria which normally live and pass their lives in your intestinal tract. The "bugs" especially favored by these particular gas-promoting foods happen to be *gas-forming* bugs.

Not all bacteria do form gases, but this particular bunch does, in the process of living their life. If *they* get a lot of their favorite foods they are going to prosper, there'll be many more of them, and consequently a lot more gas than usual, which can bloat you up and make you feel pressure in your belly. (The well known gas that comes from eating *beans* is produced in this way. Gas-type bugs like beans, it's a favorite food of theirs.)

Effect of Bacteria

These bacteria that we're talking about here don't cause *diseases,* they can't really do you any harm, and they're just eating away on some of your food and making their living that way. As you probably know, other also harmless bacteria are usually to be found in all of the other openings and on the outside surfaces of the human body. There they are, in your mouth, on your nose, on your skin everywhere, and so on. The intestinal tract, while it may seem to be internal and protected within your body, is in a medical sense considered by doctors really to be *outside* the body, and the cavity of the intestinal tract, that is, the *space* inside the tube, is in a very real sense in contact with the *outside* world. The tube is open at both ends, the mouth and anus, or at least can be and is opened frequently, so that bacteria have a ready access to it.

Well, then, we have said that vitamin C is a favorite food, or at least a favorite auxiliary food, of certain groups of bacteria which habitually form gas as one of their activities. These particular bacteria strongly favor muscle fibers of meat as their favorite food, and they can form a lot of gas from meat *without* much help from vitamin C, but if you have *both* a lot of fibered meat *and* a lot of vitamin C, you're usually in for gas and lots of it. That, of course, is why I said you should cut down on this particular kind of meat while you're on vitamin C for your cold.

Let's review again what you should go easy on: generally speaking, all meats (and fish *is* a meat) made of *muscles*. However, not all muscles are equally appealing to gas-forming types of bacteria. They just love beef and lamb, particularly if you'll grind it up (hamburger and lamb patties) so they can get at it easier. These are their absolute top favorites. They like steak too, yes, but that doesn't get ground up so well. Your teeth don't—or at least usually aren't asked to—match the butcher's meat grinder at pulverizing meat fibers. So go very easy on these kinds of foods. Ham gives less trouble partly because it's salted. Chicken is much less likely than beef to promote gas, fibered muscle though it is. Eggs and cheese are seemingly solid products that come from animals too, but they're not *fibered,* and they promote little gas. *Non-muscle* meats like liver aren't likely to form much gas either, for most people. Get down to a *starch* food like spaghetti with plain tomato sauce and you'll hear *nothing* from the gas-forming bugs. They'll be practically starving.

Again let us point out that eating beef and lamb, or indeed almost anything (remember the exceptions of buttermilk and yogurt, though) will in no way diminish the effectiveness of vitamin C in controlling your cold. I ask you to limit yourself on these foods only while you're taking vitamin C *as a treatment* for a cold, mark that statement, *treatment, high* doses of the vitamin. When you're using vitamin C for *prevention* of colds, using it in much lower doses, no modification at all of your diet is needed.

Diet Hints

There are two reasons why it is wise to limit your intake of these specially gas-forming foods (the listed meats, and also beans) while you are on high vitamin C dosage. One, you'll form less gas at the time and be more comfortable without that gas. This is really not a greatly important reason, because it'll soon be over either way. But reason number two may be important, it could be or not, so why take a chance when you don't have to? Bacteria are living things, they are a living population, which if given a special break, may be able to continue to survive for at least a while in much greater numbers than they would usually, even *after* the special break they had has been removed. Give the gas forming bugs a big break by flooding them with vitamin C and don't deny them their usual favorites like beef and lamb either, and you may be in for a lot of gas-forming bugs in your belly for some time to come.

However, such a permanent or semi-permanent change in the makeup of the bug population in your intestines (intestinal "flora," doctors call it) takes *time* to develop. A permanent change favoring gas-formers can practically never be accomplished in the 10 to 12 day length of the standard vitamin C treatment for colds. But I still want you to play it safe, so go a bit easy on gas-forming meats.

Before we leave this discussion we might just say a few more words in general about gas in the gastrointestinal tract, in case any of you are interested. This is one of the commonest complaints that the human animal has, it's just about as popular as backache or headaches. I'm not speaking now especially about people who are taking vitamin C as a medicine, but about everybody, all of us. Intestinal gas is a very frequent complaint. As I've already mentioned, a certain amount of gas should be considered normal, especially for an animal—a human—who insists on eating quite a bit of meat even though his chemical machinery is not as well designed to digest that type of food as is the digestive system of the "carnivores" (the word actually means "meat-eaters"), animals like wolves, dogs, and the cat family in all its sizes. We humans are really still "herbivores," digestive machinery-wise, and should be eating bananas and assorted vegetables, mostly.

Effects of Intestinal Gas

Not infrequently gastrointestinal gas is so bad that the doctor is asked to do something about it. Then you are liable to get quite a few tests made on you, including a set of not-entirely-pleasant x-rays called a "g-i series." The doctor is looking for such things as duodenal (the next part just below the stomach in the intestinal tube), duodenal ulcers or gall bladder trouble, and it is proper of him to do so, of course. But thinking doctors are beginning to suspect that probably the most likely of all causes for excess g-i gas is after all only a predominance in there of naturally gas-forming bacteria whose overwhelming presence has been favored by the type of diet we have been eating. One familiar example is the well known "beer belly," wherein a man is liable to have a very prominent, globular abdomen but his legs and arms don't seem unduly fat, nor his face either. This fellow isn't a really fat man, he may not be overweight at all, and the enormous belly is actually only a balloon full of gas. He's a heavy beer drinker, yes,· and the brand he likes probably has some carbohydrates (starches and sugars) in it, which are, as usual, the favorite foods of *some* bacterium or other, and this time it's another of the gas-forming bacteria. Beers and the like vary very widely in some of their components, and some are much greater gas formers than others. How good or bad they may be at gas forming always has some relation to *who* it is that is drinking them, too, we must allow, to what bacterial families he's supporting in there in his intestinal tract already.

Another not often enough considered factor relating to the bacterial flora (or "bug population") of the human intestine is how it may have been changed or modified not alone by the nature of a person's continuing diet, but also how it may have been altered when you took an "antibiotic" ("against bacteria") medicine orally, that is you swallowed it. Such powerful medicines, whose discovery and application to disease are undeniably among the high points of recent medical science are, when taken by mouth, and especially if kept up for more than a week or ten days, quite liable to change the make-up of the bacterial population of your intestine, and some of them can result in your carrying about a greater proportion of gas-forming bugs than you did in earlier times. Ideally, antibiotics should not be given by mouth at all, unless the *disease*-causing germs you are aiming to kill are themselves located in the intestinal tract. In that event, medicine by mouth is the most direct, safe, and economical way to attack the bugs. If the disease germs are in any part of your body *other* than the`intestinal tract or on the skin or in the body openings where you could reach them directly, it is usually better to get the antibiotic medicine more directly into the blood stream than by swallowing the medicine, that is, we would prefer that an injection be made into muscle (or a blood vessel). Such an injection is not going to disturb the bacterial flora of the intestine in some unpleasant direction.

Are Bacteria Necessary for Food Digestion?

Since I've sometimes been asked this, I better put in here that the bacterial populations we find inside everybody's intestines are not, doctors feel, really necessary to our digestion of food, and they're there mostly for their own good rather than for ours. On some occasions they may help to break down foods, and perhaps speed up our digestion a little, but the whole question is of no particular practical importance whatever because there isn't too much we can do about the bugs being there. As soon as a new infant takes his first food from the mother's nipple or sticks his thumb into his mouth we're off to a start on a life-long bacterial flora in the intestine. It may vary from time to time but it's yours from then on.

#5

**YOUR DIET AND DRINKING WATER WHILE
ON VITAMIN C FOR A COLD**

Mrs. Feronia P., housewife and part-time office receptionist. "Are there any special foods that will *help* you while you're on vitamin C for a cold?"

Answer: You refer, of course, to being on vitamin C for *treating* a cold. No. The very large amount of vitamin C that you need in this situation and are getting from your pills could hardly get any worthwhile boost from any amount of ordinary food that you'd be able to take in at the same time. Recall that the daily amount of vitamin C needed at the start of a cold, that is about five full grams or 5000 mg., represents 75 to 150 oranges depending on their size. How many of those 150 could you account for by eating oranges directly? But as to *prevention,* enough oranges *regularly*—and here I mean maybe only two to three per day—may be able to do something to keep you from getting colds. Remember "an apple a day keeps the doctor away"? That old wives' tale undoubtedly was rooted in what vitamin C can do to prevent you from catching a cold. And one official doctors' research study in modern days proved that it really was true that a single apple daily did cut down the chances of your catching a cold, although this wasn't a very strong guarantee.

Another question from Mrs. P: "Should you drink a lot of water when you're treating a cold with vitamin C?"

Answer: It makes no difference one way or the other.

#6
CAN YOU ALSO TAKE OTHER MEDICINES FOR YOUR COLD WHILE YOU ARE TREATING IT WITH VITAMIN C?

Edward K., 58, leather shop foreman. "While you're on the vitamin C treatment can you also take something that might have helped you before?"

"Such as what, Mr. K?" I asked.

"Oh, D_____capsules, or H____'s Quadruple Cold Tablets?"

"Did *they* help you?" I put it to him flatly.

"Not much, no."

Answer: It likely won't *hurt* you too much to take other cold "medicines" along with vitamin C, but it isn't going to help very much either. There is *no* symptom of a cold that vitamin C doesn't take care of, and no other "cold medicine" dares make that statement. The fact that every single symptom of a cold is benefited by vitamin C treatment is strong evidence that the vitamin is really getting down to a basic level and genuinely helping a cold. My patients feel that nothing they've ever tried for their colds is anywhere near being in the same class with vitamin C. No drugstore cold tablet, nor for that matter doctor-prescribed medicine either, no sun lamp treatment, no rest in bed, no steam bath, no forcing of fluids, no amount of alcohol to "kill the cold," no throwing salt over your left shoulder, or anything else now known, actually has any real effect on the course of a cold, nothing except vitamin C—and interferon, which we can't get and use in any practical way as yet.

The "cold medicines" can do nothing but make ineffectual stabs at possibly two or three among the total of eight or nine symptoms that go to make up the average cold. They really can't do anything useful, and some of them have unpleasant side effects on you, actions you *don't* want, such as making you nervous, drying your mouth, or raising your blood pressure.

Warning on Nose Drops

I particularly want to caution you against using *nose drops* at any time. Nose and throat specialists of wide experience do not favor them. Nose drops may briefly seem to open up your nose a little, but after that there is a rebound effect where the nasal mucosa swells *more* than it would have if left alone in the first place. Continue nose drops very long and you can end up with a "boggy" mucous membrane, one that tends to run something of a swelling all the time. This is a true vicious circle for your nose. Besides, there's something else that can help you open your nose, something that is wholly safe for you to use—a heat (*not* sun) lamp. You can buy the infra-red bulb at the drugstore and put it in any of your lamps which has a *porcelain* socket, which can withstand the heat generated. Put a light layer of cold cream on your nose and cheeks, and sit with your face 15 to 18 inches away from the lamp for 15 minutes. Cover your eyes and lips, since there's no point in heating *them* up. This treatment will almost always open your nose for a while. Sure, it doesn't last, but it doesn't hurt you either. Of course, there should be no call for the heat lamp to open your nose except possibly during those first 12 hours before your vitamin C takes hold, or if you've been too late at starting a successful vitamin C control of your cold.

I don't think it's necessary for me to prove to anyone that we have no good satisfactory treatment for colds readily available to us, that is, except vitamin C. Once vitamin C has had a few hours to take hold—provided always that this is an *early* cold, of course—you won't need anything else, and even *before* it takes hold, what do you have now that can really do you any good?

#7
WHAT HAPPENS IF YOU STOP VITAMIN C TOO SOON WHEN YOU ARE TREATING A COLD?

George H., 56, school bus driver. "I got along pretty well at first and figured my cold was just about over, so I quit taking the medicine after about three days. By the next morning I had my cold back again, just as bad as ever. And then it went on and lasted just as long as it would have if I'd never done anything to it in the first place, as if I hadn't taken any vitamin C at all. What do you say about that?"

Answer: You cannot stop taking vitamin C until the cold has burned itself out, unless you're willing to have it back again. If you stop short with vitamin C, or if you cut down the dose size *before* the recommended time for reducing it, you're running a grave risk of getting back the cold symptoms within about 12 hours. Once this happens, it is important that you immediately return to whatever dosage you had just been on, and which was successfully holding your cold in check. Even then it'll take you another 12 to 18 hours to get back to where you were, with the cold slapped into line again. Then proceed along with the instructions and this time behave yourself better. What George H. did, take his vitamin C well for several days and then completely stop it, I have purposely done on some occasions. This is a way of *delaying* a cold, you see, only delaying it, because you later let it go ahead and break out again, and it will then go on and run through its whole course as usual. There has never been any other known way but vitamin C of being able to intentionally delay a cold, and it can prove useful at times to be able to do this trick, even if you don't plan to continue and treat the cold the whole way through. Suppose you're scheduled to throw your two cents in at the local P.T.A. meeting tomorrow night and you start coming down with a cold. You'd like to be able to hold that cold off, at least till you've had the chance to trumpet out *your* attitude on sex education in the 4th grade. You can do just that with vitamin C.

Why would there ever be a time when you'd then be willing to go ahead and put up with the rest of a cold anyway, willing to settle for only *delaying* it for a couple of days? Well, there could be several reasons. One reason might be that you happen to be unfortunate enough to be one of that small number of individuals who can't take that much vitamin C without unduly upsetting your stomach set-up. I had one fellow who could take heavy vitamin C for about three days, but after that it wasn't worth it to him. His stomach burned him too much, though he had no discoverable stomach ulcer. This fellow was too heavy a drinker, and I think that was the reason.

I'll freely admit there may be no *good* time for you to have to undergo a cold (one that is for some reason not treatable all the way through by vitamin C). There may be no good time, but there may be a "less worse" time for you. I just want to bring out the point that you can often do some useful good for yourself without necessarily commiting yourself to a full 10-12 day course of the vitamin.

#8
VITAMIN C AND "STOMACH" ULCERS

John L. L. Jr., 24, Vietnam veteran discharged from the service because of recurring stomach (duodenal) ulcer. "Why don't I have any trouble taking vitamin C if it's an *acid*—ascorbic acid? I was told to steer clear of acids and pamper my ulcer in every way possible."

Answer: I don't know exactly why you don't have any trouble. All I can tell you is that some people with ulcers *aren't* particularly bothered by things that you would think ought to bother them. I'm not referring to those fellows taking vitamin C, I'm just telling you that there are people whose ulcers act like this. I've had only two persons with ulcers certainly *proved* by x-ray or surgery that I had the daring to try high doses of vitamin C on. I don't want to ask anyone to try anything that I myself haven't tried first, but I don't have an ulcer. One of the two I tried vitamin C on took it very nicely and one didn't. If you have a known intestinal disease we'd have to be very careful about suggesting that *you* use vitamin C, that is, by swallowing, for your colds, and we'd have to try it very gingerly to begin with in your case. I think I'd try out a few 250 mg. doses at three hour intervals some day just to see what it would do to you. Of course these wouldn't be enough to do anything to *treat* a cold, so you could make this trial any time. If you got away with it you could hazard trying a full dose schedule when you do get a cold. If you get away with that, well and good. If you can't handle that much vitamin C, you may have to settle for using it just to *prevent* colds rather than to treat developed ones, and this, after all, is really vitamin C's most useful power against colds, anyway.

#9
CAN COLDS BE TREATED WITH VITAMIN C IN SOME OTHER WAY THAN BY TAKING IT BY MOUTH?

Curt M., city highway department employee, 42 years old. "I must be one of the unlucky few who seem to get gas from vitamin C. I must admit that hardly a day passes that I don't get a roast beef sandwich in my lunch pail, and I haven't gone out of my way yet to change that, that's true. Could I take vitamin C in some other way, would it work?"

Answer: It is possible to get vitamin C into your blood stream without swallowing it, yes. You could take it by injection, directly into a vein, or into the muscles of your buttock. And it works when taken this way. This method of getting vitamin C would have very little effect on the bacteria in your intestine, one way or the other. So you could eat what you wanted and get no more gas in there than you'd have gotten anyway, without any vitamin C—or very very little more gas. *But,* who wants to take a needle every three hours? That's exactly what we had to do when we first got penicillin, at the end of World War II—we had to have a shot every three hours. Believe me, that was hateful. I myself had the connections it took to get penicillin in 1945 when it was in very short supply and the services needed more than even they had. And I also had the problem—ears—that needed penicillin, too. So I got it, and you know where, I guess. Those arrows into my rear all around the clock, the nurse jolting me awake at 3 A.M. for the next needle. Rough as it was it was worth it to block the pain of an ear infection.

But for a mere cold it just isn't a good bargain to have to take needles, even though the vitamin C could very probably be prepared so that a single needle a day would do the trick, what doctors call a "repository" injection. It's even conceivable that a single needle dose could be prepared that would cover a whole cold, that you'd need only one injection for the whole thing. That would be a horse of a considerably different color, and most handy for children. But as it stands right now, you see, there are one or two rules, half a dozen maybe, that every family physician, if he loves his profession, must always follow. An important one of these rules has always been: "The treatment must not be worse than the disease." A cold is not a very serious affliction, especially now that we have penicillin and similar medicines which can be counted upon to control and defeat the secondary bacterial infections which may follow up virus colds, and which are and always have been the real dangers in getting a cold. Having to take any great number of needles would definitely constitute a treatment worse than the disease.

#10

TINY MUSCLE TWINGES AND "ODD" HEADACHES IN A COLD BEING TREATED WITH VITAMIN C

Gary M., 16, high school athlete. "There's been all this talk about gas in your stomach, but nobody's mentioned anything else that might go wrong while you're taking vitamin C. *Are* there any other things? I had a pain in my right shoulder—it's not my pitching arm, because I'm a southpaw—along about the 9th or 10th day of the vitamin C course. I don't think I've ever had a twinge in *that* shoulder in my whole life, and I can't imagine why I should have had it this time—I hadn't done anything to the arm. It went away the next day, but I wondered about it."

Answer: The twinge was definitely due to the fact that you had a cold and you were treating it with vitamin C. In *any* cold it is not unusual for the sufferer to have a localized pain in some particular muscular location. You've probably heard someone say, "the cold settled in my neck," and he was unable to turn his head very far without it hurting a good deal. We don't really know whether some of the viruses actually did succeed in penetrating into a localized region of neck muscle, or whether they may possibly have made their way into a portion of the brain, or perhaps only into the nerve that leads to the neck muscle that we feel the pain in. (At this point we'd bet our money on the viruses being in brain or nerve rather than in muscle where they *seem* to us to be.)

A muscle pain that is due to the attack of a virus somewhere can often be recognized as such, or at least very strongly suspected of being virus-infection-caused (rather than an injury), by several peculiar features of the pain. First, there was no known preceding physical injury to the part in question, such as any kind of sprain; second, the pain has nothing to do with moving or using the muscle, it hurts when the part is lying still, resting, and is relaxed; third, the pain is quite likely to be in a somewhat unusual location, one *you* rarely if ever feel a pain in.

Well then, such virus-caused muscle sensations are expectable parts of colds for many people at some times, and they may and do occur also in colds that otherwise are being quite well suppressed (held in check) by vitamin C.

Another little oddity that you may run across during vitamin C treatment of a cold is a small headache that also seems to be a bit unusual for you. It may cover only a tiny area, say the size of a quarter on one temple, or it may be in a part of your head where it is quite uncommon for you as an individual ever to experience a headache. These headaches may be weird for you but at least they're always little headaches. They don't hurt very much and they don't last very long.

Odd muscle twinges and strange little headaches, then, are the two "weirdies" that sometimes show up in a cold being treated successfully with vitamin C. If they're going to show it'll usually be in the later part of the treatment schedule, somewhere after the 6th day, when you're cutting down the dose of vitamin C rather rapidly. They don't appear too often, but you should know about them and not worry about them. However, they do have a very definite meaning—they mean you're not getting quite enough vitamin C anymore. Increase your dose level back up to the next higher stage and keep that up for 24 hours. This almost always gets rid of the "funny." Then you can go back to the lower dose and proceed with the rest of your schedule. This will add a day to the overall length of your treatment, though. It is not absolutely necessary that you do go back up to the higher dose and have to add this extra day to your treatment, but it's being on the careful side to do so. The "funny" will pass away anyway, but not quite as promptly.

Most medicines of every type can sometimes cause certain things to happen to you besides what you principally wanted the medicine in question to do for you. Such secondary, unwanted actions are called by doctors "side effects." But we should not label the two little oddities we've just been discussing as side effects; they rather are signs that we are taking slightly too small a dose of the medicine. When vitamin C is used as a treatment for only a relatively short period, say less than two weeks, even if that be in very high dosage, as it is in treatment of colds, the only mentionable side effect that is at all likely to show up in the person taking it is the gastrointestinal gas we have mentioned.

 # 11

**A COLD BEING TREATED WITH VITAMIN C "LASTS" LONGER
THAN IT WOULD LAST UNTREATED**

Sylvia B., librarian. "You've said several times that an ordinary cold—one you *don't* treat—will last five or six days, perhaps, yet the recommended vitamin C treatment schedule requires you to take the medicine for 10 or 11, or even 12 days. How come?"

Answer: A cold being treated with vitamin C *does* last longer than it would if you let it run its natural course. There's no point in our denying that, because it's absolutely true. But you see, at the same time that it lasts longer, it is also proceeding on a very low level—all the symptoms are so slight and tiny that it's pretty hard for us to tell that we even have a cold at all. We're vaguely aware of it, we're certain we have a cold, yes, but it's so far submerged down there that it's just no bother to us. I've had only one or two people out of hundreds who hold it against vitamin C that it prolongs the whole process of a cold, because, of course, of the really remarkable effect it has on smothering your cold down to nothing.

Actually, this slowing up and lengthening of the cold is one of the most striking proofs you can give to the doubters that vitamin C really can affect the course of a cold, not in just some slight and questionable fashion, perhaps, but very dramatically indeed. Name me anything else you know of that can purposely make a cold last *longer*. I challenge anyone—physician or otherwise—to show me that *he* can *at will* make a cold *worse* than it cares to be on its own, in any manner whatsoever that he may choose, only excepting, of course, vitamin C.

You may be saying to yourself at this point, "What kind of an argument is that to make? Here he is claiming that vitamin C has a real and genuine action against the common cold, but it is a *bad* action. It makes the cold last *longer*. What kind of an argument is that?"

Well you see, if you know what you're doing you can make vitamin C's action in colds be an all-to-the-good one. Of course, any sensible person wouldn't use vitamin C to make a cold *worse*—and this can be done, I'll warn you about that again later so you don't do it to yourself. It pretty much boils down to this: do you want a typical, bothersome, burned-nostril, runny-nosed, sore-throated, sicky-feeling, laryngitis-ised, run-of-the-mill cold for six days, or will you trade that willingly for ten days of having to remember your vitamin C and having next to *nothing* else, only the rarest little subsurface hint that there is a "silent" cold slowly burning itself out somewhere within you? The people I've worked with have unanimously answered that choice in this way: they won't travel anywhere anymore without a sealed bottle of their own vitamin C with them. The bother of taking the pills, the gas that a few of them get, the "funny" little symptoms that at first seem peculiar until you recognize them for what they are, none of these nor all of them put together can swerve these friends of mine from defending themselves from colds by using vitamin C.

Why does the use of vitamin C lengthen a cold? Because the true cure of a cold still has to come from the body's own response to it, probably through the production of interferon. Vitamin C is not itself a direct cure for the common cold. It merely is a suppressor of *symptoms,* and the final cure is still going to have to come from the body itself. If you make a cold very mild by treating it with vitamin C, you actually are making it so mild that it doesn't immediately "anger" the body enough to get it started on manufacturing interferon fast. But the body's cure is only *delayed* a little, it's not done away with, and we'll get the cure finished up a few days later, and it'll be as solid a cure as ever and will also protect us against more colds for the next several weeks just as usual. And meanwhile we will have lost no time from our lives.

For the umpteenth time, I'd rather you miss getting a cold at all than for you to get one and have to treat it. The more you learn about this little monster the more likely you are going to be able to evade it completely. My "trainees" miss out on a lot of colds, more than half of what they used to catch, in fact. *If* they goof—and sometimes that is truly unavoidable—then they treat.

#12
HOW SUCCESSFUL IS VITAMIN C AS A TREATMENT FOR CHILDRENS' COLDS?

"This is Mrs. M., speaking for Billy M., ten years old, 4th grade. Billy came home from school on a Friday afternoon with a cold. He hadn't had it at breakfast time that day. I put him right on vitamin C, not so much for himself alone as for the three younger ones. By the next morning, Saturday, he was so much better I saw no reason to keep him in, and let him out to play. But I made him report back into the house every three hours, and he did pretty well at that, taking into account that I was sure he'd show for lunch, which he, of course, did. I didn't let him have his usual Saturday favorite meal though, because it is baked beans and frankfurts, which are both on the not-recommended list. All he said about the cream cheese and olive sandwiches was, 'Is that all you made, Mom?' And being hungry again, he reported back in at about 3:30, too, so I got the medicine into him pretty regularly.

"About the same thing happened Sunday, too. I let him go to Sunday School that day, and by Monday morning he was still feeling top drawer so I packed him off to school as usual. Of course I saw to it he got his vitamin C at 8:15 just before the school bus left. I gave him his vitamin C pills for the day in an empty matchbox, and wrote out and put in the box the times when he was supposed to take them, at 11 o'clock, and again at 2. They shift classes in his school every hour on the hour, so that would fit well. He didn't want the teacher to know he was 'sick' and he promised me he'd take the medicine for sure by himself. But he has to bus so far that he can't get home for lunch, so I had to put him on his honor about the pills. What do you suppose happened? He was feeling so good that he could see no sense in taking medicine, so he didn't. He seemed so well when he got home from school I just couldn't believe his cold hadn't gone its way, and I myself let him out of what would have been the 5 o'clock dose. But just as we were sitting down at the TV for the 8 P.M. news, who do you suppose pops up with, 'Gee, my nose is running, Mom'? Well, I got vitamin C into that boy before they were through the commercial, that's how fast I moved. Then I shook him awake every three hours through the night, setting my alarm to do it. The next morning I reviewed with him just exactly what he was to do that day—when he was to take the pills.

"Can you possibly guess what happened this time? He lost the matchbox somewhere. Has anything ever exasperated you like a little boy who loses things? They can't give you a hint as to how they did it, so you have nothing to work on to see that they don't do it again the same way. This time I had a harder time getting him into good shape with all through the night vitamin c than I'd had the first night. In fact, I was hard put that Wednesday morning as to whether I should let him go to school, or make him stay home where I could keep my eyes on him. He was in pretty good shape, but would he stay that way? Well, I'll ask you into a koffeeklatsch if you can guess what my Number One son did this time. No, he hadn't misplaced the box again. He was just bending over the drinking fountain in the hall when along comes another boy, and he wanted to know what Billy was doing. Billy said, 'Taking my medicine.' 'Are you sick?' the other boy asked. Whereupon what does our little hero do? He throws his matchbox across the hall, and the five pills fly in every direction. No, he's not sick and no kid is going to think he is.

"Doctor, I've taken enough of your time and you wouldn't believe the rest of the story anyway. I let him go to school Thursday because he wasn't too bad, just a little runny-nosed, and when I had him at home I kept up his vitamin C, but at school I didn't even try it anymore. But the teacher sent him home early anyway Friday because his throat was sore again and he was blowing his nose every couple of minutes. I watched him like a hawk on Saturday and Sunday but this time the cold just didn't respond to vitamin C. It just went right on as it pleased. By this time I was down to a 250 mg. size dose with Billy, but it seemed to do no good at all. When Monday came I couldn't let him go to school, because his voice was all hoarse and he said he felt sick. Remembering your instructions not to keep up with vitamin C if it's obviously not doing what you want it to, I stopped it altogether. By Tuesday his nose finally began to dry up, even though he wasn't getting any vitamin C anymore. But still I think this was one of the *worst* colds he's ever had. And before the rest of the week was out Ginnie and Dick came down with colds too."

Answer: Billy's unfortunate story has several valuable lessons in it for us. *First,* vitamin C in the only readily available dosage form we now have easily at hand, that is, tablets that need to be taken every three hours, is not very satisfactory to use to treat a cold in smaller children. This is not because the medicine isn't effective in children, but rather because we just can't count on kids of this age to take the responsibility for getting the vitamin C into themselves with the regularity that is absolutely required if the medicine is to work well. Every day Billy had a different reason for not taking his vitamin C, and for some of these reasons we as adults with all our experience in life have to sympathize a little with him, that's true. Anyway, children vary a great deal in the degree of responsibility that they will show, even for themselves, so we cannot make any hard and fast rule about who is too young to take vitamin C successfully for a cold, or who is mature enough to surely be able to do so and succeed nicely at it. Experience does suggest that a normally bright child of 12 or over, especially a girl, usually can be counted upon to keep up her vitamin C schedule nicely, and usually gets good results from this treatment for her cold. For children under that age the results just don't justify recommending it for them as a routine thing, if *they* have to be responsible for a major share of the dose schedule.

Experiences with Children Taking Vitamin C

Where I have had children under very close supervision, vitamin C has worked as well as it does in adults. If a parent was responsible for every dose without exception, the medicine did very nicely. I did not cut the doses of vitamin C very much from the standard adult size doses because I wanted to make sure that vitamin C could work as well in children as it does in adults.

If a child weighed at least 100 pounds I used full adult doses. Only if he weighed in the 60-75 pound region would I use a lesser size dose, and this still amounted to about 3/4 of the adult size doses. I've used vitamin C on only a handful of children six and younger because as the treatment stands—such frequent doses being necessary—I doubted whether on the whole this treatment would be worth the effort.

In making this evaluation I also always kept in mind several important points. (a) The worst parts of a cold, especially for children, are the secondary bacterial complications, bronchitis, mastoid, that type of thing. These can almost always be treated nicely these days with penicillin and similar medicines, so that it is not absolutely necessary to hold the basic underlying virus cold in check so as to prevent the first appearance of these complications, as it would be if we didn't have penicillin, etc. (b) I feel that, compared to adults, there is a considerably lesser urgency that children, particularly the younger ones, must be kept forever ready to perform their every day's share of the world's labor without a single lapse. Ten years from now—indeed one month from now—it'll make no significant difference that little Johnny missed that Tuesday and Wednesday in shopwork class, or even in American History.

When we can determine a consistently successful schedule for the use of vitamin C given in long-acting capsules, and most particularly if we can develop a one-time-injection dose of vitamin C that will cover a whole cold, then we can rightfully take a different look at the use of vitamin C to treat colds in small children. Until then, good sense suggests that insofar as treatment of a developed cold is concerned, we should limit this very effective but oh-so-critical-to-administer medicine to those whose personal responsibility will mean certain success in the use of the treatment—adult size *responsibility,* whatever your age may be.

Billy's history points up a *second* important lesson for us, too: it is most important that you use *enough* of the vitamin to ensure getting good results in your cold. Viewed overall, Billy's mother considered this cold of his to have been *worse* than if it had not been treated by vitamin C at all. By "worse" she meant principally that the cold had been much extended, and that several times it broke out again with symptoms that had already once disappeared several days before. Billy's cold lasted longer than it should have, and it came and went several times. This is exactly what happens when a cold is treated with vitamin C but *not enough* vitamin C, and had nothing directly to do with his being a child of ten. The same in-and-out type of a cold will show in any adult who slips into taking vitamin doses that are too small, or who begins to take his doses too infrequently, even if individually they are still of the right size. Now while it is true that there *is* some small individual difference from person to person in what size doses of vitamin C he will need to control a cold, compared to some other person, still *most* people, the great majority of them, will need a dose of at least a certain size if their colds are to remain continuously suppressed, that is, controlled down to a not-bothersome level. So I first had to determine if there was *any* amount of vitamin C that would successfully hold colds in check for say some 95 percent of the people using that dose. This done, I next had to find out what the *smallest* amount that would do this successfully would be. It was finding out what size dose of vitamin C would be the *minimum,* the smallest amount of vitamin C that would *consistently* hold a cold in check for *most* people that took me some five years and more to get through. Well, I did that, and I also learned in the process that a dose still smaller than that might often hold the colds of perhaps 50 percent of cold victims in check, and even smaller doses still would sometimes work for perhaps a quarter of people suffering from colds. But these lesser rates of success for vitamin C in a cold—a quarter or a half treating well with a particular dose, anything less than a 95 percent success—wouldn't be good enough. Who knows, at least in *your* first trial of the treatment, if *you* are one of the ones who could get by with a smaller dose than the standard? If you couldn't get by, if your cold wasn't controlled, you'd immediately stamp this method of handling a cold as still another flop in a field historically full of failures—useless treatments, things that really didn't affect a cold at all. You should be a *success* in your first treatment of a cold with vitamin C, if my win-you-over beat is to go on, as they say in the ads.

Why "Full" Vitamin C Doses?

There is perhaps an even more important reason for you to be given a dose size of vitamin C that will surely be *successful* at treating your cold. If a dose is *not* going to be successful, it unfortunately often turns out to be not just merely useless to you, but *harmful* to you. This is in the sense that too small a dose, but still a dose of vitamin C, will often result in your cold lasting *longer* than usual and at the same time *being just as bad as it usually is* for all this extra time, too. Let us make this very clear: "half" doses of vitamin C—by which we mean any less-than-sufficient doses of the medicine—will give you the *lengthening* of the cold process that we have already learned is always the inevitable accompaniment of using large amounts of vitamin C to treat a cold, but at the same time half doses *won't* give you the complete smothering of the cold that a "full" dosage level brings with it, and which is what you want. A "half"-treated with vitamin C cold is longer than a non-treated one, and just as bad as usual anyway.

TABLE SHOWING HOW DIFFERENT DOSAGES
OF VITAMIN C WILL WORK IN TREATING DEVELOPED COLDS

(We are *not* talking about *prevention* of colds here, and we are assuming that we are getting started with treatment in the first 24 hours, as we always must. Also, we are here referring to the *total* daily amount of vitamin C used, and we mean that amount at the *beginning* of a cold.)

A. "Small" doses of vitamin C
    (daily total 250 mg. at beginning)
        Result on symptoms of cold: nothing
        Result on duration of cold: nothing
    (The cold behaves as if no vitamin C at all were being taken: this size dose is good only for *prevention.*)

B. "Half" doses of vitamin C
    (daily total 2½ - 3 grams (2500-3000 mg.) at beginning)
        Result on symptoms of cold: usually nothing, no good—
            only a few persons will benefit at this dose level
        Result on duration of cold: lengthened, lasts as much as
            four extra days, all of it as bad as usual completely
            untreated cold

C. "Full," standard doses of vitamin C, as suggested in this book
    (daily total 5 or more grams (5000 mg and up) at beginning)
        Result on symptoms of colds: excellent, very good
            control for nearly everybody
        Result on duration of cold: lengthened, again lasts as
            much as four extra days, but symptoms extremely
            mild or invisible, all the way through

"Standard" Doses

Where did the "standard" doses come from? As I say, they were worked out by actual trial and error over some 8-10 years, first on me personally, then on the rest of my family, then on my earliest official research group of patient-friends, and finally further tested on an expanded group of many other people of all sizes, ages, types, and locations. Most of these people lived in the northeastern U.S., but some additional ones lived in the South, and several in Hawaii. Then other physicians all over the country and in several foreign countries contributed *their* experiences with treating colds by using vitamin C. Everywhere, and everybody seems to respond in similar and satisfactory fashion to vitamin C for their colds. If they get enough vitamin C, get started early, and keep it up, they get very good results. If they don't, they don't. It's that simple.

The doses that I have found to work out nicely for 95 percent of people are what are being given to you in this book as the recommended (adult) doses. Incidentally, still larger doses do *not* usually succeed in turning the 5 percent of people whose colds weren't well controlled into successful treatments; these were failures for reasons other than dose size, but most of them can be converted to successes also—at the same dose size. We'll discuss these people later, and show you what particularly to watch for if you happen to be that rare person—that one out of twenty—who doesn't get an excellent control of his cold right off by following the standard instructions. Suffice it to say I have yet to personally meet an individual whose colds will not respond to vitamin C when it is properly taken.

To be on the safe side why don't I just recommend that you use even larger doses of vitamin C than are suggested in this book? Would they work? Yes, they would. Here's why I don't suggest that. The doses of vitamin C that you *must* use if you wish to hold a cold in check successfully are already very high doses indeed, and the use of so much vitamin C is absolutely *not* completely free of danger, even though a great many people at large, and entirely too many physicians, too, still incorrectly think that it is utterly harmless although perhaps largely useless for you to take so much vitamin C.

The overall view of most of the medical profession today on the use of vitamin C—for *any* purpose—is still that (1) a very small amount of it (what we have called the "vitamin" level, perhaps 70 mg. a day, rather than the "treatment" level, 5000 mg. a day or so or even more) will do you all the good that can be done by *any* amount of this vitamin, and, (2) that any excess of it you take (over that 70 mg.) will probably do you no harm, but will surely be a waste of your money, that's for certain. More than once I have heard of doctors expressing themselves on this latter opinion in these words, describing a patient of theirs who for one reason or another (not always colds) likes to take a lot more vitamin C than the doctor thinks can possibly do her any good: "She has the most expensive urine in town." They mean by this that all the extra vitamin C is really only being passed directly through the patient's kidneys, where it is promptly strained out of the blood stream and immediately disposed of without doing you any real good.

The actual fact is that while the vitamin C *is* being excreted by the kidneys (yes, that's true) it meanwhile is at a very high level in your blood plasma, and if you happen to be harboring a kind of condition that vitamin C can benefit, such as an active cold, it *will* be benefited, whereas a very much lower ("normal") amount of vitamin C in your blood would be too little to do that disease any good. For a doctor to use as an argument against *any* medicine the fact that it may soon be strained out of the body by the kidneys is nothing less than ridiculous, because a great many other of the "wonder" antibacterial drugs that the same doctor would not give up using at any price are, especially when taken by mouth, handled in exactly the same way by the kidneys. That's exactly why so many of the modern miracle medicines have to be taken every four to six hours around the clock when they are being taken by swallowing pills.

When a doctor gives as a reason against the use of substantially large doses of vitamin C that this extra ascorbic acid will all too soon only be passed from the body in the urine, he is demonstrating to one and all his complete ignorance of the fact that this substance, ascorbic acid, *is* in *large* doses, a *medicine,* in addition to still being in small doses a "vitamin" proper.

Fortunately, many more physicians *are* newly learning what vitamin C can do, often in diseases where there is no other successful type of treatment whatsoever at this time. This vitamin is by no means a panacea—a cure-all for everything—though, and we must keep our heads about vitamin C just as we should keep a moderate and reasonable position on everything else in life if we can.

Why Graduated Doses Are Recommended

Why don't I advise you to take the full beginning dose of vitamin C all the way through your cold? Would it work? And wouldn't it be easier than having to make these dose reductions from time to time? Of course it would work, and it might be easier too, but it would be taking an unnecessary and uncalled for risk. A good physician always uses the *least* amount of a medicine that will successfully accomplish what he is trying to get done for his patient, and, again, he doesn't even use that *if* this treatment would be worse for his patient than the disease is. Since the common cold is not a very serious condition, any acceptable treatment for it has to be a pretty trouble-free kind of treatment. One good way to keep vitamin C for treating a cold trouble-free is to not use any more of it than is really needed. Since as a cold progresses less and less vitamin C is needed to keep it in check, it is advisable for us from the point of view of maximum possible safety to cut down the dose size as it is possible to do so. It's true that that makes for a nice balancing act on your part between taking enough vitamin C and not taking more than is required. But if you'll follow the schedule we have given in this chapter you're not likely to run into trouble.

On a few occasions I *have* directed a person to simply take the full 5 grams a day of vitamin C and continue at that same level for 12 solid days. But since I wouldn't want him to go on doing this indefinitely later by himself I did not tell him what it was that he was taking, only that it was a "special cold medicine" he could get only from me. And, of course, it worked fine.

I cannot say too often that in spite of all the cautions I keep throwing at you about your steering clear of taking too much vitamin C, you can hardly get yourself into any *permanent* trouble with vitamin C no matter how much you take of it, if only you'll stop dead with it after no more than the 10 to 12 days of the suggested treatment for colds. It's *long continued* treatment at *high* dosage—dosages much greater than 500 mg. a day—that can switch your intestinal bacterial flora to the "gassy" type. This won't happen if you use even astronomical doses of vitamin C for only a short stretch, or if you use only small doses even if they are taken over very extended times, from one's year end to the next.

Billy's cold *was* made worse than it would have been without any vitamin C treatment at all, and this *was* because his mother, once having decided to try it, allowed herself to slip into letting it be carried out carelessly. But this most likeable lady did learn her lesson, and to this day she has never forgotten it.

13
WHAT HAPPENS IF YOU CUT DOWN ON YOUR DOSE OF VITAMIN C TOO FAST WHILE TREATING YOUR COLD?

Roger B., 50, jack-of-all-trades. "Yesterday was my third day on treatment, and I had only a little hoarseness left. Everything else was gone, so I cut my dose to 400 mg. This morning I could feel I had a throat condition. What should I do now?"

Answer: You are a scamp. You reduced your dose, you descended to a lower level of vitamin C dosage *while you still had a noticeable cold* symptom. Never do that. A "little hoarseness" is still a symptom. It means you can't hope to cut down your dose yet. Anyway you're not supposed to cut down on the beginning dosage until you have *completed* three days at that high level. You'd only completed two. I'll bet if you had finished three full days at the 625 mg. level you'd have had no trouble when you dropped to 400.

As a matter of fact, once in a while you are going to find it necessary to go an extra *fourth* day at the beginning 625 mg. level. This would be if (1) you weren't quite totally symptom-free at the end of your first 72 hours of treatment, even though you had carried it out superbly, *or* (2) if halfway into the 4th day of treatment, which is the first day you had cut down to 400-450 mg. size doses, you began to notice a return of symptoms. In either of these events, take another day at the full, beginning dosages—625 mg.

It is practically never possible for you to shorten up on your vitamin C treatment by cutting out one of the *first three* days, that is one at the 625 mg. level. Sometimes you can get away with dropping one day from the next stage down, the 400-450 mg.-per-dose days, that is days four through six of your treatment. But usually the safest days to try to drop from the schedule are near the end. If you end up with a 10 day total treatment rather than a 12 day one, and if it was a successful one all the way through, the days you skipped will usually have been some of those from the 8th day on; if you had tried to skip a couple of early ones you would probably have had to restore them and add on an extra one, too, as a "punishment."

Rather than trying to get by too quickly with a lesser dosage, it's more important for you to use enough vitamin C to turn the trick when you need it, and then later, at the end of the treatment, to get off the medicine completely and promptly as soon as you no longer need it at all. Now I know, Roger, that *you* have nothing particular against taking vitamin C. I know that you like what it does for you. But I must again stress to you that the hallmark—the certain proof—of proper vitamin C dosage in colds is *always* a satisfactory suppression of the symptoms. Anyone who is not prepared to take the required amount of the medicine to accomplish this is better off not to take any at all.

14
HOW A WOMAN'S MENSTRUAL PERIODS MAY AFFECT THE DEVELOPMENT OF A COLD AND HOW THEY MAY AFFECT THE VITAMIN C TREATMENT

Mrs. Mabel B., 34, hairdresser. "Doctor, I was getting a cold. I was sure I was. The inside of my nose itched and it was maddening to feel the drops starting to roll down inside there. But I had a stiff line-up of appointments that day, and I had only 400 mg. of vitamin C in my pocketbook with me at the shop, that was in case somebody were to sneeze at me, of course. I took it, but I knew it wasn't enough for even one beginning treatment dose. I just couldn't get out of there until after 6:30 because a woman had to be set just before she left for the opera. Anyway, by the time I got home I forgot about taking any vitamin C because I seemed to be better by then. My nose had stopped dripping. But a couple of days after that I blossomed forth again with a real lulu of a cold. This time I treated it with vitamin C and got rid of it just about as usual when I use the medicine. What I don't understand is about that day in the shop. Was that just some sort of allergy? Did one of the hair solutions annoy me, do you think, or was one of the customers wearing perfume that bothered my nose? It certainly seemed like a cold. I thought I was in for it, for darn sure. And I did get a honey of a cold, only those two days later. What do you think, Doctor?"

Answer: I thought, and it turned out I was right, that Mabel B. must have started her regular monthly menstrual period just about the time her cold broke out for the second time and ran its course. It was obvious from her story that the first incident of runny nose in the beauty salon had really been a beginning of a cold, but that something had intervened to stop it, at least temporarily. I'd noticed this kind of thing on several occasions before. Women of menstrual age, which usually runs from about the age of 12 or 13 to about 50, will often show a striking ability to delay a just-caught cold if it happens to them just a day or two before their menstrual period is due to begin. This delaying power—which acts very much like a good course of vitamin C—usually lasts two or three days only. It starts a day or so before the actual period begins and lasts only through the first day of the period itself.

Then it is lost, and the cold will make a reappearance and continue on from wherever it was before it was brought to a temporary halt. Only an early cold can be stopped thus by an approaching menstrual period; one that is three or four days along at the beginning of the monthly does not seem to be affected at all. That behavior too—a late cold being unaffected—reminds one of the way vitamin C operates. The stalling of a cold by an approaching menstrual period is probably accomplished by some hormone (active body chemical in the blood stream) that is being specially produced at that particular time as part of the monthly period. We just don't know whether the actual way in which this hormone accomplishes its trick of delaying a cold is similar to the way in which vitamin C does the same thing or not. But in any event, a woman in this age group should be aware that such a thing can happen, and can stand ready to expect a return of her cold in several days. During the hormone-protected period she will find that it is not necessary for her to take vitamin C to block her cold, but she may want to be prepared to use it to carry on the treatment once the hormone protection is over.

#15
MY BEST OPINIONS ON THE USE OF THE VITAMIN C TREATMENT FOR CHILDRENS' COLDS

Mrs. Dorothy A., surgical nurse. "Doctor, it isn't quite clear to me just how you think a *child's* cold *should* be treated."

Answer: I think that as much as we can we should try to spare smaller children from catching colds in the first place. At this point in medical development we haven't got the ghost of a chance to do this very often, but we should do what we can. Quick vitamin C control of the colds brought into the home by older family members will forestall at least some of the smallest fry's colds. Scrupulous attention to household hygiene (dishes, etc.) once a cold has invaded the home will block a few more colds. If we lose all these bets, as we sometimes surely will, and the little ones do show a cold, put them into bed in a room by themselves, mainly to keep the other kids away. Do anything that seems to comfort them and that you're sure won't hurt them, such as chest rubs, extra TV, and reading stories to them. You're just trying to ease their way through the unavoidable and do no harm in the process. If an older child, a parent, or an aunt or uncle has had a cold recently and thus probably has his own immunity, try to assign that person and no one else to caring for the little victim. This will help a lot to stop the spread of the cold to other as yet unaffected family members.

If you as the mother are the only available "nurse," and come down with the cold yourself, be quick to control it by vitamin C to keep it from jumping to the other children through you.

I think that for the smallest offspring—eight and under, I'd say—it's probably much the best to let nature solve their colds at its unmeddled-with fastest, that is, *without* vitamin C, at least in the pill form we have to use it in at this time. Keep always on the alert for the secondary bacterial complications that are the real dangers of childhood colds, and if you have any doubt as to whether these ear, throat and chest involvements are about to threaten or not, turn that responsibility over to your family doctor or pediatrician. That's what he's there for.

However, when things have cooled off again and none of your brood has a cold at the moment, don't be too quick to be sold on the idea that a tonsil and adenoid operation for each child will drastically cut down on the number or severity of what you consider his too-frequent colds. I'll tell you the truth—sometimes T & A operations make a child's cold situation *worse* rather than better, and it is just not so that this operation should be done practically as an accepted routine on every child, cold problems or no. That's not medicine, it's only salesmanship.

16
USING VITAMIN C IN TOO WIDELY SEPARATED DOSES

Dr. Whitten V., 50, "I took 2 grams of vitamin C q.i.d. but it didn't help my cold."

Answer: ("q.i.d." is doctors' lingo for four times a day, that is, every six hours.) Although this comes to a total of 8 grams a day your doses were too widely spread at those six hour intervals. Even large doses of vitamin C fall precipitously in the blood plasma by the end of three hours, customarily. Of course a *continuously* high blood level of vitamin C is necessary at least in the opening stages of a cold. If you don't keep it up there *all the time* you'll get no good results.

A COMMENT ON THESE PROBLEMS OF VITAMIN C
TREATMENT OF COLDS

We have, then, in this latter part of our present chapter, just been skimming our way through an examination of the fortunes of one person after another as they face up to the realities of having to entertain that very unwelcome guest, the common cold, and as they use vitamin C to help them do so. We have carefully studied how this vitamin-medicine can assist us against colds, and if it has seemed to you that many of our examples have been only another *problem,* another difficulty that attends upon our using vitamin C, that is only because it is not necessary for us to concern ourselves very much with those things that go along quite well by themselves. So you have not been hearing so much about how well things *usually* go, but in actual fact vitamin C treatment of a cold—provided always that it be *early, sufficient,* and *well sustained,* according to the principles we have outlined—is nearly always a very smooth-flowing, satisfying, unquestionable success that has few false turnings and that will please you to no end. Those of our example cases that are problems are relatively rare of occurrence, and they have been given an undue prominence here far beyond what their infrequency could properly deserve, in order to make it as easy as possible for you to be able to straighten things out for yourself, and go on to success should you happen to meet up with one or the other of these relatively rare birds.

In thinking back over this chapter we should perhaps again recall to mind that a good, successful vitamin C treatment of a cold, one that will turn out very nicely as viewed over the long run, is still going to need about 12 hours to work in the first place before you will be noticing your first improvement, the first notable controlling of your cold symptoms. From then on, *no* symptom should ever get out of line again, and if it does it will almost certainly be *your* fault, because you skipped a dose or more, or delayed a dose, or cut down the dose strength too quickly. Whatever your flaw, if it is allowed to continue, or be repeated, you will pay for your lack of care by a return of some of your cold symptoms. If this happens you will then be forced to weather another stretch of some discomfort, because a cold symptom once returned usually cannot be forced back into disappearing a second time in less than some 15 to 18 hours, no matter how precisely you may pick up and adhere to the treatment schedule this time around.

The cardinal sins of an unsuccessful vitamin C control of the common cold are too late, too little, and too short. Too late a start. Too little a continuing dosage. Too short a treatment over all. Watch out for all three and you'll be okay.

6

The Controversy About
Vitamin C

Vitamin C has already been used by many people for 15 and even for 20 years for the treatment of their own personal colds with very excellent results.

Why is it then that *you,* the reader of this book, are only now hearing for the first time about the remarkable powers that vitamin C has against the common cold? Certainly it's not because you yourself haven't asked scores of times, "Why can't they find something that will cure a simple little cold? How come they can cure a terrible thing like tuberculosis, and stop in its tracks the Black Plague that killed a quarter of all European population during the Middle Ages? They can even prevent the horrible paralysis that polio used to bring only a decade ago, and yet they haven't the tiniest suggestion for us about what to do for a common little cold, not the slightest idea of anything that will really help it at all."

Well, now that you've come this far in this book, you recognize that most of the formerly very dangerous infectious diseases that we can now handle nicely these days are caused by *bacteria* rather than by viruses, and you know that conquering bacteria is ever so much easier than winning battles against viruses. You interrupt me right here and you say, "Polio is caused by a *virus,* what about that? If you can solve that with a vaccine, why

don't you do the same for colds?" Well, polio can be caused by
three different viruses, but only by these three, and polio vaccine
actually is made to act against all three of them.

It is a general truth that vaccines may be remarkably
effective, but to work they have to be very specifically designed
toward a particular, limited target. As we know, colds can be
caused by possibly a hundred different viruses. It would be ever so
much more difficult to make a cold vaccine that would work
against all these invaders, but there's a still more important point
against it. Polio is a disease which once haα, you usually don't
catch again. You are permanently immune to it. That's what polio
vaccine does, basically. It gives you a very mild, controlled form of
polio. Your immunity is thus stimulated and once you have
established this immunity you are protected forever. But colds
don't work that way, of course. Your immunity to them is a
short-lived matter of only weeks. So a cold vaccine is not worth
the trouble.

All right, so you have asked plenty of times for something to
help you with your colds. Why didn't you get vitamin C?

WHAT DOCTORS SAY ABOUT VITAMIN C FOR COLDS

The principal reason for not being treated with vitamin C is
that doctors, the ones who could put a solid stamp of approval on
this treatment, and are the logical ones to tell you about it, have
not as a group ever been completely convinced—as yet—that
vitamin C definitely has a good effect on colds at all. All along
there have been numerous individual doctors whose own experiences with the medicine, both on themselves and on their patients,
have absolutely convinced them that vitamin C's powers against
colds are unquestionable. But by far the majority of doctors still
remain unaware of vitamin C's remarkably good effects on colds.
If you ask one of these fellows—and the chances are that your own
doctor is one of them—what can really be done for colds, he'll say,
"If you want the truth, nothing." If you ask him what about
vitamin C, he'll shake his head, "No, there's nothing to it."

Now I'd like you to clearly understand that your doctor is
not misguiding you on purpose. He remembers he's heard some
mention of vitamin C from time to time in connection with colds,

but it was vague, and he honestly thinks that it was finally decided
that vitamin C was useless against colds. Nor is your doctor using
vitamin C for his own colds, holding out on this secret and keeping
it from you.

The first thing you must realize is that most doctors just
aren't very much interested in colds or the treating of them. They
have a great many far more important and serious diseases to
concern themselves with, so the average doctor rarely gives a
moment's thought to the subject of the common cold. If you
knew the tremendous amount of new information about really
important diseases that's being thrown at doctors these days, and
the terrible labor it is to try to keep up with it and still be able to
do something for patients at the same time, you'd find it hard to
criticize your own physician for his limited concern over an old
chestnut like the common cold. And what happens when our
favorite family doctor does snatch a minute somewhere and picks
up a professional medical journal to try to keep himself abreast of
the latest medical developments? Most all of the reports in these
scientific magazines are usually put together by the researching
doctors, the doctors who are still studying and trying to make new
medical advances to get us a little further along the way. The
researchers usually have no ordinary patients or practice to
command 101 percent of their time, so *they* can do experiments
and write articles to be read by the practicing doctors. Well, then,
here we have our own doctor looking into the professional medical
publications in his effort to stay abreast and what does he find
there? Not one article in a thousand will say anything about the
common cold. It just isn't a glamorous target for researchers. It
isn't one of the things that are "in" these days in medical research.
It won't generate a huge grant of money, and it does take money
and lots of it to conduct research in most cases.

So as far as vitamin C and its use in colds goes, our doctor is
left just where he already was some 12 to 15 years ago. During the
1940's and 50's there *was* a substantial flurry of interest among at
least some doctors as to whether vitamin C—and a few other
medicines—could really benefit a cold, or whether they could not.
The general public, of course, has never lost interest in the
common cold, and has continuously hoped for a really effective
treatment for it. The interest the medical profession showed for a

time had its basis, as did the public at large's also, in the hundreds, even thousands, of incidents that people, including doctors, had noticed over the years about the apparent good effects *at times* that foods that contained vitamin C seemed to have had on colds. Things like "hot lemonade being good for a cold," or "an apple a day keeping the doctor away."

And so for a few years right after World War II quite a few medical articles were still appearing that reported on tests of the use of vitamin C against colds. Sometimes other medicines were combined with vitamin C in a test, and sometimes it was used alone. In most of the experiments the testers were more interested in what vitamin C might be able to do to *prevent* your getting colds than they were in whether it could successfully treat a cold you had already caught. The reason for this was that few of the researching physicians even dared to hope that vitamin C—or indeed anything else—could possibly help an already developed cold. Nearly everybody just took it for granted that nothing was going to help in the *treatment* of a cold that had already appeared, so the only big questions remaining were simply—could vitamin C guarantee that you'd get fewer colds, or at least see to it that they would be milder ones if you did catch them?

RESEARCHERS' REPORTS ON VITAMIN C

Some of the researchers who reported their work in the medical journals at that time felt that their tests had definitely shown beyond any reasonable doubt that vitamin C used on a regular basis did reduce the number of colds that would have been expected to occur in a particular group of persons, such as a class of college students, and often tended to make a cold milder too. But in these tests colds were by no means completely done away with, and some of the students individually seemed to have gotten nothing out of taking the vitamin C; they had as many colds as ever, and just as severe ones.

Other researchers felt that *their* particular work had made it equally clear that vitamin C had no real value whatever in the prevention of colds, and did not make for either fewer colds or less severe ones. In other words, there was a variety of opinions expressed pro and con among experimenting research physicians as to the possible value of vitamin C against colds, though each considered his own studies to have been well organized and properly carried out, that is, worthwhile and fully dependable.

The upshot of all this work was the general conclusion among most doctors that vitamin C had had its chance to be fairly assessed as a possible useful agent against colds, and, like everything else, had pretty much flunked this test. Surely, there were occasional hints here and there that vitamin C had helped some people, but overall the picture wasn't nearly good enough to justify recommending vitamin C for colds, even halfheartedly. The result was that almost all research work on the common cold, vitamin C treated or not, pretty much ground to a halt, in the United States at least, around 1956-58.

This then was the background that went so far to form our average doctor's impression that vitamin C has no genuine value in colds, and it is true that until very recently he's had no very convincing reason to modify his stand on this subject. So the medical profession at large had come to the general conclusion that vitamin C has no useful powers against colds, and it had come to this conclusion on the basis of what it considered good and valid evidence, that is, well-conducted research work by trained experts in this field. In the profession's view, any of the general public who continue to put an obviously unfounded faith in vitamin C as a good treatment for colds are at the least misguided if not incurably ignorant, and any maverick physician who still insists on continuing to trumpet vitamin C's anti-cold values has certainly blown his mind, if he's not an outright charlatan. Actually this isn't a very much overdrawn picture of the medical profession's attitude.

Yet the truth is that vitamin C *does* possess a remarkable, unequalled power to suppress the common cold even when it has developed; a power to hold all parts of it in check and this no matter which particular virus may have caused it. Vitamin C also has extremely impressive credentials as a preventer of colds for you, as we shall be seeing in detail in chapters to come. A few doctors, and amazingly, many of the not-medically-trained public, too, have steadfastly held to their own positions on vitamin C through the years—that it most certainly *is* a splendidly effective deterrent of the common cold. They held to this certainty not at all on mere blind faith, but based on what they had themselves experienced time and again, success with vitamin C.

THE DIFFERENCES OF OPINION IN MEDICAL CIRCLES
ABOUT VITAMIN C

How can it be that the majority of the medical profession can think one thing, and yet a handful among them, along with a part at least of the admittedly medically-untutored public, think something else that is entirely different? Who's the wrong one? How can all those *doctors* be wrong, especially when they took into account so much well-performed research work? But on the other hand, how can the other side—the pro-vitamin-C people—be so sure of what *they* say? Are they just deluding themselves, *hoping* it's true?

The answer is that neither side is wrong. They're both right—*in so far as what they're talking about goes.* You see, the pro-vitamin C people (vitamin C *for* colds) are talking about one thing, and the anti-vitamin C people are talking about something quite a bit different. The antis are talking about using relatively *small* doses of vitamin C, while the pros are talking about tremendously larger doses. I will be the first to agree that vitamin C has no visible effect against colds *if* you are going to use it in what we have called "vitamin"-size doses, say 70 mg. total a day (which is the current official government "minimum daily requirement," "M.D.R."). You have to use vitamin C in "medicine"-size amounts if you wish it to show its power against colds, and this, you remember, calls for up to *five thousand* (5000) mg. daily for cold *treatment* (at the start), and even for *prevention* as much as 1500 mg. is needed to cancel out an obvious cold contact (we'll be discussing this in the next chapter). You need a probable minimum of 250-500 mg. daily even when you're using vitamin C most of the days of your life, for a long-term, wide-range prevention of colds. When the antis say vitamin C won't work, they mean 70 or 100 mg. won't work. When the pros say vitamin C *will* work they mean 500 or 1500 or 5000 mg. will work.

Every bit of the research done in the 1940's and 1950's made use of considerably smaller doses of the vitamin than it really takes to show consistent good results against colds. So it's not surprising that the experimenters came to the conclusion that vitamin C didn't help colds very much. But actually all they had really done in their research studies was to show that *so-and-so many* milligrams of vitamin C didn't accomplish such and such a good against colds. And indeed these researchers often said precisely that—that *so-and-so many* mg. hadn't helped. It was often not the fault of the test experimenters themselves that *other* doctors, and non-doctor medical reporters, both of whom had been only *reading* the reports of the research work and had had nothing to do with the. actual performance of it themselves, went on and expanded a very specific statement that say, *100 mg.* of vitamin C had been given daily to 2000 college students, and it had not cut down the frequency of colds in this group at all, into a generalized conclusion that vitamin C does nothing to prevent colds, period. When you make a flat, unmodified, undecorated statement like "vitamin C cannot prevent colds," what you are actually saying at that moment is "vitamin C cannot prevent colds *no matter what size dose of it is being used,* and *no matter what the conditions of the use may be, no matter how it may be taken* (oral or by needle), and *no matter if you happen to be standing in the Sea of Tranquility on the moon,* and no matter anything and everything else, too."

It is not scientifically acceptable for us to proceed to such a wide generalization as this example we have just given, that "vitamin C (flatly) won't prevent colds," if that sweeping assertion was based merely on experimental work that had been limited to one little corner of a big problem—the tests confined themselves only to relatively tiny dosages of vitamin C. Such a tiny slice of the possible "whole pie" can fairly be taken to shed light only on that particular little section it was dealing with, and cannot be widened to form a safe conclusion about what would happen under other circumstances and in areas it was not dealing with, that is, considerably larger doses of vitamin C. Once in a great while one of the vitamin C medical research reports of this period did come perilously close to hitting the mark, musing briefly about maybe trying more of the vitamin sometime, but then they always backed off from actually testing the larger dosages that would shortly have pinned together as the truth all that wealth of hints that had already surfaced, both in the medical "literature" (the whole body of professional medical magazines, both present and past) and in the "outside" world.

THE AUTHOR'S PERSONAL RESEARCH FOR A COLD CURE

It was in 1959 that I myself became even more interested in finding a successful treatment for colds than I had been before. And at that time I found the situation to be pretty much as we have just described it. There were many hints and suggestions in circulation that vitamin C *could* do something against colds, that it had at least some value in *preventing* them, and there were even one or two scattered claims in the medical literature that vitamin C could do something even against an already developed cold, that is, *treat* it.

But in general the whole subject of vitamin C's possible powers against colds was very much muddled up. The "cons", or anti-vitamin C people (often doctors), were sometimes prone to make rather tactless *personal* remarks about the "pros," those who favored vitamin C as a treatment for colds, or indeed, believed it was useful for *anything* other than the disease *scurvy*. It wasn't too hard for the antis to say these things since some of the pro-vitamin-C people were making really fantastic claims of all kinds for vitamin C, for which claims they had not the slightest shred of a scientific basis at all. So it was easy to label *anybody* who thought vitamin C was good for anything beyond scurvy as a "faddist," a "food nut," or in the case of a physician, a "quack." But, as we have already pointed out, all through this period there continued to be some of the general public, and always a few physicians, too, who "kept their heads" about vitamin C, who had a pretty clear idea of what it would do, and still didn't allow themselves to entertain any illusions about what it *couldn't* do.

These sensible "moderates" were, unfortunately, lumped in with the faddists and quacks, and even M.D.'s themselves found it very difficult to get the medical profession in general to sit down and even *listen* to what they might have to say. The losers were the medical profession, the general mass of doctors themselves, as well as certain of their patients, because with the passage of time it is now becoming more and more clear that vitamin C can have a favorable effect—in some cases can actually save lives—in certain *serious* virus diseases for which there is at present no other specific treatment whatever available. I want to make it clear that this seeming certainty that vitamin C can help to cure several dangerous, possibly fatal virus infections other than colds has not yet been *proved* according to the techniques that the medical scientific world demands as proof, and rightly so demands.

But I will say this much on this subject right now: if I, or anyone I was responsible for, were to show up with virus hepatitis (liver infection), virus pneumonia, virus-caused encephalitis (infection of the brain), influenza, or polio (this in spite of polio vaccine or lack of it) or any of several other virus-caused infections easily recognized by doctors, *I* would lose no time in getting huge amounts of vitamin C, as much as eight to ten *grams* (8000 to 10,000 mg.) daily into that sick person, by intravenous injection for the rapidest possible usefulness. In such a situation there is absolutely nothing to lose, and everything to be gained, because these are *serious* diseases—I'm not talking about a mere cold now—and we have no other treatment for them at this point. In these diseases, as in the common cold, it is vitally important that the medicine vitamin C be started *early,* and kept up religiously. In such serious situations it should not be taken by mouth until the condition is obviously much improved, and even then not by mouth if our victim can't stomach pills yet.

THE SEARCH FOR FULL VITAMIN C POWER

After looking over the vitamin C-and-colds situation as it stood in 1959, I had felt that a deeper examination of the whole question was probably still justified. The idea that vitamin C might help colds didn't originate with me, of course. That idea had come from long ago in folklore. But what I did say to myself was, if vitamin C can do *something* for a cold, maybe more of it will do more and better. I didn't see too much risk in trying more of this particular vitamin, although I was well aware that it was possible to get *too* much of some of the other vitamins, particularly vitamin D. Neither did I forget a favorite phrase of doctors, "*Enough* of anything can poison you—even water."

I started right at home on myself, and in general I increased vitamin C dosages in each cold I caught as each increase in the medicine gave me better and still better results. I always recognized that all the gloomy conclusions of those other doctors merely meant that vitamin C hadn't been very helpful against colds *at the dosages they used,* and that's all that these studies had meant. After about three years' worth of colds and much jockeying around with the dosage of vitamin C, I finally arrived at what are pretty much still the dosage levels and timing schedules I've been recommending to you in this book. By then I could do just about what I cared to with my own colds. I could knock a cold down and keep it there until it died without ever bothering me, or, on the other hand, by playing around with vitamin C, sometimes using it and then taking it away again, this cycle over and over again, I once managed to purposely string out one of my colds for 27 days.

By now all four of my nearby relatives were also controlling their colds very nicely with vitamin C, all of us succeeding with it in very much the same way. All the starch had been taken out of our colds. But even a consistent and surprisingly good success in treating colds was far from enough if it was in only five individuals. Perhaps there was something special about the individual members of so small a group as this. Maybe *most* people's colds *wouldn't* dry up and behave as well on vitamin C. I had nothing so far in the way of good "controls," people suffering with the same colds at the same time and being given only faked vitamin C placebos instead of the real medicine. Neither had I done my work so far in a double-blind fashion, or even single-blind for that matter. (In single-blind, at least my cold-medicine-taking subjects wouldn't know whether they were getting vitamin C or maybe only chopped sawdust, even if *I* did know.)

Since very few animals can catch human-type colds, and the few who can would necessarily have to live a very unhuman type of life in their laboratory cages if *they* were to be the subjects of a vitamin C-and-colds test, I jumped directly to continuing my studies on humans exclusively. It's true that chimpanzees can catch colds, but chimpanzees are scarce and costly. Suckling (baby) hamsters also will take the common cold, but they're quite distant from the human species. This brings us to what was really my strongest reason for not bothering with animal experiments. Since he has stated this reason so very neatly, I'm going to lift the words of one of our clever Chinese-American medical researchers—we have more than a few doctors of Chinese-American descent in scientific research in this country, and their work is of a high order. These are Dr. Chang's words, practically as he gave them out, for your benefit.

He said: "In virus infections the attacking virus and the host cell (*your* body cells) *work together as one unit*," and even if it has been shown that a medicine *can* stop a particular virus in a certain kind of test *animal*, "it may make a lot of difference *which* animal you had to use," meaning (and here's the part of his statement I like best of all), "if we wish to have wonder drugs against human virus-caused diseases, we cannot escape being used as 'guinea pigs' *ourselves* before any great progress can be made toward getting these medicines."

ANIMALS AND HUMAN GUINEA PIGS

So in this particular situation of the common cold not only were even chimpanzees and hamsters pretty much out, they'd probably have been a mistake, too. Anyway, by now I'd already had considerable personal experience with very high dosages of vitamin C on myself and other humans, and I had a pretty good idea of what this vitamin can do, on both the good and the bad sides. And, of course, very importantly, vitamin C was not a newly invented medicine by any means, and it had already been used for many years by millions of people, and sometimes in even greater dosages than I was going to use in my expanded studies. So I went ahead.

I easily found myself some more willing people-type "guinea pigs," and one of the largest vitamin manufacturers in the country made up tens of thousands of special capsules for me. Actually there were four different capsules, because I was also testing out another medicine thought to be possibly helpful in colds, as well as vitamin C. (Incidentally, that one proved completely useless.) Two of the four types of capsules contained some vitamin C and two not, but all of them looked exactly alike, and not a bit like ordinary drugstore vitamin C; they were large orange capsules, not round white tablets.

My new subjects were instructed exactly how to use the

medicine when a cold began, and to keep in frequent touch with me by telephone, but they were *not* told that they would actually receive four different kinds of capsules (only one at a time, of course) nor were they told what would be in any of the capsules. They had to promise to continue with the full treatment schedule even if it were doing absolutely nothing for them, which indeed happened about half of the time, because half of the time the capsules they got purposely contained only milk sugar or the other medicine I was testing, which, as I have just said, had no useful effect on their colds. When my people were using either of the capsules that had no vitamin C, their colds were affected not in the least, either way, and once they'd gotten through these unmodified colds in the usual no more than five to seven days, I'd then let them off the hook from taking the rest of the schedule. When they were taking capsules which did contain vitamin C and their colds were being well suppressed, they were required to go through the full schedule. Each person received each of the four kinds of capsules during some cold or other of his, usually each "medicine" several times, because most of these people stayed with me for from three to five years, and during that length of time they had anywhere from 7 to 20 colds apiece.

As often as I could I would treat two or more people in one household with different capsules at the same time, because it was highly likely that they had the "same" cold, and this would give me a chance to see what different medicines would do against the same virus. This was, of course, one of the ways I sought to put controls into my tests and thus give them more validity. In some cases I was fortunate to have all four different capsules being used in one family at one and the same time for what was almost surely the "same" cold in all of the household. Since I was conducting the tests in proper double-blind fashion this time, I wasn't myself allowed to know which person got exactly what, but I could ask my secretary to give me four different medicines for a particular family.

Fortunately for this kind of research purpose, if for no other reason, the common cold *is* a kind of disease that does recur fairly regularly and is often very much the same in its reappearances. Combine this with the fact that colds don't kill their victims, so that they will live to have to face up to yet another cold on some future day, and you will see that we have another very nice type of control for our tests. Remember that a "control" is a *person,* a person whom you fake giving a medicine to, in order to help show that another person with the same disease who got real medicine and gets well was cured *by that real medicine.* One individual person can serve as his *own* control if he will oblige us by getting the same disease from time to time, further oblige us by surviving so that we can still have him at hand, and third and finally, we also want him to oblige us by letting us give him different medicines in the succeeding attacks of the disease so that we can compare these medicines. All this can be done nicely in the common cold—if we're polite to the fellow and don't wear out our welcome.

So I had managed to set up a test of the medicine power of vitamin C against colds, and it was a test that would finally show whether this vitamin could successfully stop a cold or whether it couldn't. Whatever my test was going to show, it would do so fairly and accurately, because the test had been designed properly, and would be carried out properly, according to standard scientific requirements, including the use of controls, placebos, and the double-blind technique. To my knowledge this was the first and only time that *any* medicine has ever been *proved* to affect the course of a common cold favorably, proved in the prescribed manner.

Actually, that's about all I did that hadn't already been done by other people. I really did it not to prove anything to the medical profession, but principally to satisfy myself. As I've said, a few other doctors had long been treating colds with high doses of vitamin C and doing very well at it, and so had quite a number of not medically trained people at large done the same thing for themselves individually. But too many people still wouldn't believe that it worked. Buddy, *now* you better believe it!

In all, some 45 different people took part in the rigidly supervised portions of my tests, and in the long run not one of them turned out to be unable to get good results in his colds by taking vitamin C *if* he behaved himself according to the instructions. Since then, many other persons have tried the treatment also, *not* under any test conditions, and I don't know one of them who didn't work out well, too, again, *if* he closely followed the schedule.

THE TEST OF CONSISTENCY

In order for any treatment for any disease to be acceptable, it has to *consistently* bring good results. That is the key word—consistently. A treatment need not succeed every single time, in 100 percent of the cases, because the best treatments there are just don't have records quite that good, whether they're medicines, operations, physical therapy, x-rays, or throwing salt over your, left shoulder. But an acceptable medical treatment has to succeed in a very large proportion of the times it's used. Of course, the more serious the disease, the smaller the percentage of success a treatment for it will have to have to please us. Since the common cold is usually a quite mild disease, any acceptable treatment for *it* must have a very high rate of success, and additionally, this treatment must pose very little danger of its own.

There *are* individual persons who can get pretty good control of their colds using somewhat less vitamin C than I am recommending in this book for *you* or who can get their colds burned out in a day or two less than the 10 to 12 days of my standard treatment. If you are such a person, you're going to have to find it out for yourself, and I suggest you use the full standard treatment quite a few times first before you experiment in this direction. And sometimes for almost anybody, a particularly mild cold may clear up more quickly and require less vitamin C than usual. But if we are going to look at a sizable assortment of colds in a sizable number of people, actual experience shows that we have to ask them all to take the full recommended amounts of vitamin C for each and every cold they wish to treat. Only then do we get a satisfactorily high rate of success in treating colds—something like 95 percent good results.

A question from Wallace B.: "Wouldn't still higher doses of vitamin C give you even better results?"

Answer: In the common cold, no. I've tried this out on many occasions. You just don't need more than five grams (5000 mg.) a day (to start). You don't get any more out of it with more than that. But you do need that much, or mighty close to it.

"But Doc, I was talking to a fellow the other day who says he has some instructions that advise you to treat your cold with 1500 mg. of vitamin C every hour for ten doses, and then 2000 mg. every two hours for another 12 to 24. And that would take care of the whole thing—just a day and a half."

Answer: I know about that suggested dosage schedule, and I've tried it out a number of times. Of course it works fine at first, because there is plenty of vitamin C there, more than enough. But most of the times I've used it, both personally and in others, the cold is by no means over with at the end of 36 hours, as is suggested. You still have to go on for some days with more vitamin C if you want to keep the cold down until it's burned out. Furthermore, you don't get to use any *less* vitamin C from the end of this sky-high dose during the first 36 hours than you would normally have to use if your first 36 hours had been only at my recommended 625 mg. every three hours level. Nor do you save any days of treatment either by beginning vitamin C at these astronomical doses. You still have to treat the cold just as long. It really isn't surprising that a mere 36 hours of vitamin C, no matter how much of it you may take, won't completely banish your cold for good, ordinarily. Once a cold has developed, made its appearance, you've got viruses there, and lots of them and what is finally going to do them in is not vitamin C but the body's own defenses. Whether we want to call this defense by the name "interferon" or not, it takes *time* for it to develop. This usually takes more than *48* hours, not 36 for your body even to begin developing its own defense against colds. And this would be in an ordinary, *untreated* cold.

Remember that taking a lot of vitamin C for your cold, though it beautifully simmers everything down, also makes it take *more* time than usual to fully work up your natural defenses against colds. A 36 hour treatment no matter how sky-high won't "cover" you until the body is ready itself to take over the defense against the viruses. We're going to need a lot more than 36 hours, then. So you needn't expect that you're going to be very likely to be able to get a quick and *completed* cure by *any* kind of very short-term treatment regime, vitamin C or not, astronomical dosages or not. And even if it did work, and worked very well, it wouldn't be all to the good because if it cured you that fast you wouldn't get enough time to work up your usual short-term immunity to the next cold in line, which, though it is only a temporary resistance, is definitely worth something. This limited immunity must be *earned* and this can be done only by your passing through the *whole* of a cold in some sort of manner, that is, either entirely untreated, or suppressed by vitamin C. If you *could* completely squelch a cold in a total of only 24 to 36 hours, as here promised, the usual several weeks' resistance would not be gained in so quick a process. Without having earned this exemption-for-a-time, you would remain constantly at the mercy of every cold virus you ran into. You might be in for a new cold every few days.

THE MEDICAL COMMUNITY'S ATTITUDE

After my professional report to doctors on vitamin C treatment of colds had appeared, I received a great many letters from physicians in different places, and also many from interested members of the public at large. Many of these letters told me of good success in treating developed colds with vitamin C. But numbers of others reported somewhat less than satisfactory results, or very poor results indeed. It was most interesting for me to see that those who reported good results were almost without exception using quantities of vitamin C that amounted to at least five grams a day or, sometimes, very considerably more than that, and that their dose timings were also fairly close together—only rarely more than three hours apart. On the other hand, those who were getting the poor results were usually using no more than three grams a day, and most of them very much less than that amount. These experiences, then, tallied very neatly with my own completely independent findings.

Question from Amelia H. and Polly P., two veteran summer vacationers to Europe: "Doctor, we saw vials of vitamin C tablets offered on the counters of drugstores in France, advertised specially for colds. There was the same thing in Spain, too.''

Answer: Yes. You see, in some European countries the rules about medicines aren't as strong as the laws we have in this country. Sometimes that's bad, but at other times it can be good. What you saw were "effervescent" tablets of the vitamin, sometimes with as much as a gram (1000 mg.) in a single tablet. They're effervescent because making a medicine bubbly will usually fool some people into thinking it's better than if it just sits there quietly in the glass. You may swallow a little easier, that's true. The instructions with these vials of vitamin C tell you to take what will come out to about four grams a day, and that *is* enough to simmer down some people's colds, but it'll miss a lot of others. And the instructions don't tell you to take vitamin C long enough either. However, it's interesting that you noticed this in your travels. It's another indication of how widespread the conviction is among ever so many people in many parts of the world that vitamin C is a worthwhile way to get at colds. In spite of the old saw, 50 million Frenchmen *can* be wrong, but this time I don't think they are.

In this country vitamin C took a terrific clobbering from all those pessimistic research reports of more than a decade ago, but in parts of Europe they've gone ahead with vitamin C and gotten some good out of it, although their recommended dosage schedules fall somewhat short of what is actually necessary for consistently good results, as I have said.

CAUSATIVE VIRUSES

Question in a letter from Dr. W. B., virologist (physician specializing in the study of viruses in the scientific laboratory): "Doctor, you don't know which the actual causative viruses were in your series of vitamin C-treated colds, do you? And you don't know for a fact that vitamin C will work against *every* virus that causes a cold either. Isn't that so?"

Answer: You're right. In doing my own cold tests I at all times treated only naturally-caught colds, just as they happened to blossom out in my patient-friend subjects. I feel that intentionally giving a cold to a person by squirting into his nose virus-carrying infectious nasal discharges from a person with a cold already, while it sounds scientifically thorough, may not come close enough to the exact details of how a cold is spread in nature. Therefore, you may not be able to get an honest estimate of the value of a certain medicine against colds, or of the dosage amounts of it needed, if you are going to test it against colds caught in an unnatural manner.

We must of course admit that the researching doctor who does cause a cold to be artificially passed from the victim to a new subject does thereby have the advantage of knowing exactly which of the one hundred cold viruses has caused a particular cold, and hence what a chosen test medicine or dose of it has been able to do against that specific common cold virus. But if you were sufficiently interested in this information—which specific virus was at fault at this time—you would also be able to identify it by taking it from the victim after he has caught his cold in the natural manner. Admittedly you might have a tough time finding enough individuals who just happened to catch the particular virus you might be currently interested in, if you weren't interested in all one hundred. This is because if you use only naturally caught colds you have to take "pot-luck" on which viruses are the criminals of the moment. I myself wasn't too interested in this end of it, identifying specific cold-causing viruses, because I already knew that vitamin C *must* work against almost all of them, maybe all, because it *had* been working all over the country for years, and so it must have run into many if not all of the possible cold-causing viruses.

I won't go so far at this time as to insist that vitamin C must be defined as a true anti-viral agent, even one of some broadness of spectrum (meaning "effective against many more than a single" virus; "useful against at least some sizable assortment of different" bugs). But I will flatly assert that that set of symptoms which we call a cold clearly can be made to bow to vitamin C in a very large proportion of instances—*if you know how to do it.*

HOT LEMONADE FOR A COLD

Question from Virginia Z. F.: "Now that you've been concerning yourself with vitamin C for so long, Doctor, can you fit some of the old wives' tales like 'hot lemonade is good for a cold' in the whole picture? Apparently you feel there was more than a little truth in many of these sayings. Just how correct were they?"

Answer: There have been literally hundreds, perhaps thousands, of hints and observations made in the wide-open domain of society at large, not all of them necessarily in the immediately recent past either, suggesting that vitamin C did have a useful action against the common cold, to some sort of degree at least. As my interest in this field deepened, I was quite impressed to find how very frequently a person who had never had a chance to work up any particular scientific background will step into his local drugstore often in some remote crossroads, and order a bottle of vitamin C, "because it's good for colds."

It now seems to be true that a remarkably large proportion of those "tips," "hints," "guesses," "suggestions," "observations" or whatever you want to call them that the public had about vitamin C and its value against colds *were* correct, at least in general terms. As soon as we came to understand what sizable doses of vitamin C have to be used if we wish to successfully *treat* rather than merely prevent a cold, and how accurately these doses have to be *timed* if we want the treatment to work well, we could then see *why* it was that those observations that people had made had sometimes seemed to be true, and at other times didn't seem to hold water at all. It was because to get vitamin C to work well enough so that you could see it working you had to have used *at least* a certain amount of it (often a lot), and it had to have been taken at a specific time in the whole set-up. Understand that and you can see how a great many of those long-recognized "hints" about vitamin C and colds do fit neatly and honestly into the whole "picture," Virginia, to use your word. Pieces of jigsaw that made so little sense when scattered at random on the table now are seen to have a true place in the completed picture. Now that we can see it all, they make good sense.

7

How to Keep from
Catching a Cold

Part 1: Your Protection Against an Obvious Cold
You Cannot Avoid

Vitamin C—and a lot of understanding on your part—can often keep you from catching a cold which you might otherwise have had to put up with. Marvelous as it is to be able to suppress a developed cold successfully, it is even better if you can evade it completely, and not even have to treat it at all. Even if you are now a past master at the tricks of using vitamin C against a developed cold, it's really better for you if you can completely get out of having to take the large amounts of this medicine that are required to hold a cold in check. That's a lot of work, and it takes a lot of days when you compare it to *not* having to do it at all. My friends who took part in our cold studies with me and became expertly trained in both the natural behavior of colds and in the use of vitamin C against them, these people now catch fewer than half the colds they averaged in the past, and most of them are just as pleased with that accomplishment as they are with their being able to successfully control a cold that has somehow sneaked past them, as is still going to happen from time to time.

In this chapter we're going to talk about how you can protect yourself on a specific occasion from picking up a cold from a person who very obviously has one. (In the next chapter we'll discuss what you can do for yourself on a year-round basis to greatly cut down your chances of catching any cold at all at any time, whether or not you happen to run into people who clearly have colds.)

It is usually possible for you to avoid catching a cold from a person who plainly has one, even if you cannot get out of his way, and even if he sneezes directly on you. This protection against a specific cold contact can almost always be accomplished by using vitamin C taken in a big enough dose at just the right time. We may, if we care to, call this the "interceptor" dose of the vitamin, since it cuts off a particular attacking virus' one chance of being able to establish a foothold in your upper respiratory tract. If you will take vitamin C right at the very time when you are exposed to somebody's active cold, you're just not going to catch *that particular cold* from that particular person. This, of course, means that you're specially taking vitamin C at a time when you don't have the cold as yet, visibly. Of course, it hasn't developed yet, because you were just given it. It's also true that you *may* not even *have caught* a cold at all at this point. But *if* you have caught one then and there (and *don't* take vitamin C) you're not going to know that you have caught it; you're not going to know until two to five days from then. If you find it out only then, that you did catch the cold—and that's the only time you *can* find it out—you're too late. You've missed your chance. Now you'll either have to put up with the cold, or treat it with the full treatment course, both of which choices are not as good as having been able to skirt around the cold somehow. However, if you do take vitamin C and take it properly at this time of contact, it's true that while you're never going to know whether you really *were* handed a cold or not by that sneeze (because it'll never develop) neither are you going to blossom forth with a full-blown cold even if you *were* handed one. So if you're wise you'll see to it that you get an interceptor dose of vitamin C at every obviously dangerous contact. And even if you are already on a regular daily ration of vitamin C the year round, you'll still specially take the interceptor dose to cover your meeting with this hapless possessor of an active virus.

HOW VITAMIN C HELPS GUARD AGAINST COLDS

Now in general, vitamin C used in different ways can do three valuable things to help us against colds. It can

(1) Force an already developed cold into submission (if it's no more than 24 hours old)
(2) Greatly reduce the number of colds you catch over any extended period
(3) Absolutely protect you from picking up a cold from a specific, obvious contact—what we're talking about just now

The first of these, vitamin C's ability to push any new but genuinely developed cold below the surface, is probably the most impressive of the vitamin's three powers against colds. For one thing, it's a valuable action that you can get without having bothered to do anything else in advance, that is, either to consider the active cold contacts you might have run into, or to be taking the vitamin on a year round protective basis with great regularity. You can get something from vitamin C even if you never bother yourself at all unless and until you've really burst out with a cold in all its glory.

I would never minimize the importance of power #2, vitamin C's ability to cut down the number of colds you catch over a period of say several years, no, I'd never downgrade that, but it does call for a very faithful taking of the medicine over a long time, and any even mild breaks in the faith are liable to be rewarded with a real cold. So, in my personal opinion, *the* most noteworthy service of vitamin C against colds is action #3, protecting you from a specific obvious infectious contact. This action, which as we have said is to be the principal subject of this chapter, provides a most valuable help to us at practically no risk whatever, and with really very little effort on our part, too. Sure, this is only a short-term prophylaxis (a preventive value lasting for only a few hours), but what a lot of value the interceptor dose can be for us.

Your First Protective Step

Here's how we do it: Within no more than an hour after

someone with a cold has sneezed at you, coughed nearby, breathed in your direction, or whatever it was, get 600 to 750 mg. of vitamin C into yourself. (You may take it immediately after this happens.) Take a second dose of the same size very close on the head to three hours after that first dose. That's all there is to it. You won't get that cold.

If you're going out for the evening and want to protect yourself, take the first dose at home just before you leave. Then you'll be able to walk untouched and apart right through the crowd of coughers. Take the complementary second dose on your return home, and you will almost certainly have escaped trouble.

Now some comments. If you're already taking vitamin C every day anyway as a long-term protection, take those regular doses just as usual also. If you are a regular user of yogurt or buttermilk, and can foresee the likelihood that you may have the occasion to want to be able to use the interceptor doses in the evening, then skip the yogurt for that day. Finally, if you want to be ready to be able to use this two-dose set of protection at any time it suddenly becomes necessary, you will have to make a habit of carrying that small amount of vitamin C with you at all times. While it's true that you have about an hour's safe leeway to get the first part of the dose into yourself, I find that if you don't take it instantly at the very time of the offending sneeze, while it's fresh in your mind, it's terribly easy for you to forget in the next few minutes all about your having been sneezed at, and continue to forget it way past the safe point. Of course you need not carry your interceptor vitamin C with you when you have recently passed through a cold and are convinced you still carry some resistance from that encounter. If a person's immunity to the next cold in line, the immunity he earns by having passed through a cold, is usually good for about six weeks, then I usually advise him that he's not at all likely to be able to catch another cold under any circumstances for probably *four* weeks, to be on the safe side. During that month there's little point in his carrying, or in taking this specific protective two-dose set of the vitamin. He doesn't need it.

Vitamin Insurance

Now how can I possibly say that taking a simple little

two-dose set of vitamin C prevented your catching a cold, when you most likely didn't even pick one up on that sneeze? Well, you'll notice I didn't say *that,* exactly. I said, *"If* you were unlucky enough to pick up a cold at that encounter, you won't get it if you take the two doses as instructed." Even considering your degree of resistance, the number and vigor of the viruses blown at you, and so forth and so on, most encounters with an active cold *won't* give you one. A good guess as to what proportion of such meetings-up with an active cold sufferer will succeed in bestowing the viruses on you is less than one-third of such meetings. (When strong viruses in substantial numbers are directly forced into your nose by a needle, with a rifle-like accuracy much better than a sneeze, even then only about 1/3 of the "targets" catch the cold in this kind of experiment.)

But, you see, the point is *some* such meetings between the virus and yourself *do* take, and I don't mean one time out of a hundred. It's a lot more frequent than that, I'd say possibly once in six tries. So over the course of time a certain proportion of the contacts between yourself and a series of cold sufferers, a certain proportion of the sneezes, coughs, etc., blown your way *will* succeed in giving you colds at least at intervals, if you're the cold-catching type at all. Particularly in the situation where you have not developed a cold at any recent time—for whatever reason that may have been—and thus have not gained the four to six weeks' immunity you usually earn against a following one it might be presumed that you would be a continuingly juicy target for colds viruses. Yet if you use vitamin C faithfully enough in this two-dose protective fashion for obvious contacts—and in this way only, *not* regularly day in and day out, too—you rarely get any cold that you would then have to go about either actively suppressing or submitting to without protest. Unquestionably at least some of those contacts must have been ready to infect you, and must have been cancelled out by those mere two doses of ascorbic acid at exactly the right time.

Perhaps I should go on and explain a little further why there's so little doubt in my mind that vitamin C can work so effectively to protect you from catching the cold that might have arisen from your specific meeting with an active cold sufferer at one particular time. To be of much value, this too had to be proved scientifically with controls to substantiate the real truth of it. It wasn't an easy thing to do by a long shot, but I think we did it.

The protective character of the two-600 to 750 mg.-dose set of vitamin C against a particular obvious cold contact was established in the first place, and can only be safely confirmed in the following manner, which is what we (myself, my office assistants and family members) did, many times: at some time during the "cold season," those of us who had had no colds for at least eight weeks (and therefore were very likely susceptible) absented ourselves for five days from all contact with any other humans by going to a remote private camp. If at the end of the five days we still had no colds this meant we hadn't caught a cold *before* we went on our little retreat (because the maximum five day incubation period had passed safely with no cold developing). Then we returned briefly to a "society" full of colds, that is we spent six to eight hours in the office with many patients with fresh colds. During this office stay we sometimes *asked* the patients with colds to sneeze or breathe at us, and then some of us took the recommended two 600 mg. doses of vitamin C, and others didn't. We then immediately withdrew back into the privacy of the camp, again for another five days, this time every one of us separate from the others in an individual cabin. Those of us who had taken vitamin C during the contact period in the office practically never got colds within the succeeding five days, but those who had *not* taken it often did, though not in all instances.

Using this procedure, any colds that did develop must have been caught during the few hours we were in the office, and the prevention of the ones that didn't appear had to have come from the single two-dose set of vitamin C that we took there. As I have said, we were purposely *not* taking regular preventive vitamin C daily through the time of these tests.

As is obvious, you can't take vitamin C if you don't have it with you. A "graduate" of my class in vitamin C once reported how he handled this oversight under difficult circumstances. He'd been dragging himself through the ups and downs of the National Forest in New Hampshire starting the last week of a very hot August, and the last thing he'd been thinking about for months was getting a cold. But suddenly one afternoon as he was taking advantage of one of the few chances to be *lifted* someplace, he realized

he'd boxed himself in, literally. Here he was trapped, riding the
Cog Railway to the summit of Washington during the weekend
right after Labor Day. The coach was full of first-week-at-school
sneezers—and, more's the pity, the windows in these new model
cars *don't* open. He was in for it for sure, and mighty unhappy.
There was no escape, and he knew there wasn't going to be any
vitamin C at the Tip Top House. Or was there? He had it! Every
trail lunch ever put out by the Mountain Club, jelly-bread-on-
store-white sandwich and third-rate chocolate bar notwith-
standing, every one of those little brown bags never failed to
include an orange, too. On top, he quickly spotted a troop of
climbers and proceeded to corner the citrus market on the "Top
of New England," at a high 50¢ per unit. Everything else was
sky-high up there, why not oranges?

"How many did you corral, George?" I asked.

"At 50 mg. a fruit, which comes to a penny a milligram, Doc,
ten was still a bare minimum, wasn't it?"

"Well, of course," I reminded him, "maybe you wouldn't
have gotten a cold anyway."

"After *four* months you think not? It was worth the feeling
of security to me, Doc," George claimed. "I had more trail to do,
and I wanted no trouble."

IF YOU CATCH A COLD EVEN AFTER TAKING
A PROTECTIVE DOSE OF VITAMIN C

We must clear up another point that has sometimes come up
for discussion. A question from Miss Doris: "I took 750 mg. of
vitamin C shortly after someone sneezed in my face, and another
750 mg. three hours later, just like you said, but I got a cold
anyway. That shows that vitamin C will not prevent *all* colds,
doesn't it?"

Answer: No. While the two doses of vitamin C taken as stated
are almost certain to protect you from picking up a cold from that
particular sneeze, the blood level resulting from this set of two
doses alone will only stay high enough to protect you from all
other contacts for perhaps six to ten hours overall. You have no
protection from any other cold contact that you run into before

or after that six to ten hour period of protection. You must keep in mind the following two points: first, as you know, the incubation period of a cold is commonly anywhere from two to five days, and second, while a cold is infectious only during a limited period of its history—usually the first 48 hours of its being visibly there—this period of infectiousness sometimes seems to begin a few hours *before* the first apparent cold symptoms. We've said that before. This means that sometimes it is possible for you to catch a cold from a person whose own first cold symptom will not appear for several hours yet, that is, the contact really responsible for the cold you're going to get two to five days later can be hidden from you. Putting these two facts together, it means that under the conditions of ordinary life where you have a whole series of contacts with many different people, it is not usually possible for you to be able to connect any particular cold with any specific contact with absolute certainty.

   Question: "How can you ever protect yourself then?"

   Answer: Generally speaking it is *not* necessary to remove yourself completely from society, which would be impossible for most people anyway, to enjoy the protective benefits of vitamin C to be taken only in this non-regular, just-when-you-see-an-obvious-contact fashion. This is because *most* of the colds that can infect you *will* be obvious to you, and if you will cover every visible contact with a two-dose set of vitamin C, the number of colds you'll get over a long period, say four to five years, will be strikingly lowered. (Your record will probably be even better if you also routinely take vitamin C daily during the nine-month "cold season" each year.)

   I think that it seems very likely that a dose of 600-750 mg. taken twice may be more than is needed to cover you from a cold contact. Later experience suggests that as little as 400 mg. only *once* within an hour of the contact is sufficient. But since during the actual controlled study process described we were at that time using two 600 mg. doses, that requirement is the sole dosage we have certainly proved to be effective. Since you're going to be taking only two doses at the most for this particular purpose, I have recommended you take 600-750 mg. size ones just to be on the safe side.

   To close this chapter, here's a question I wish nobody would ever ask, because it's impossible for me to give you any encouragement on it. But we must know the whole truth. The question: Let's say you haven't had a cold for two months. Suddenly somebody sneezes and sprays you with a cloud of what you're sure are viruses. The circumstances are such that you just can't get *any* vitamin C in either medicine or natural fruit form for say 12 hours after the sneeze. Of course, you're not going to blossom forth with that cold before an additional 36 hours at least, more likely not for another two or three days. Is there anything you can do to stop that cold? We can assume the viruses have made it inside the cells. They won't be back out again for a while. Can we do something?

Answer: That was a beautiful question. The answer is an ugly two letter word—NO. I call that stretch "the helpless period." I've never found it does any good to take vitamin C at this time. If you *did* catch it, you're in for it. You'll have to treat it when it blossoms out, or put up with it this time.

8

How to Keep from Catching a Cold

Part 2: Year-round Protection for You

By far the greatest number of people who have been using vitamin C in the special hope it will give them some help with their colds have been taking the vitamin in rather small doses (in the range of 250 mg. daily), and they've usually been taking this regularly every day, often the year round. The main thing they hope for from this is that they'll catch fewer colds, and secondarily they hope that the colds they still do catch will turn out to be milder or shorter than they would be otherwise, or both of these things.

I have no doubt whatever that many of these people *have* actually received at least part of this reward they wished for from vitamin C. I'm not so sure that the colds they still caught were always necessarily milder, nor necessarily shorter. Comparisons of this sort are terribly difficult to prove out with a proper degree of scientific certainty. But when you look at most sizable *groups* of regular vitamin C-takers, the fact that overall, as a *group,* they are getting fewer colds, seems unquestioned. Some individuals among them may not seem to be any better off as to the number of colds they still get, but the group—yes. I have received a great many letters from various schools and other sorts of organizations, and any time there are at least 20 people being considered, and the routine dose of vitamin C is at least 250 mg. daily, that group is, as a group, suffering "fewer colds than before." Now right away the doctors will start saying that that's not a "controlled" experiment; it means nothing, it's just their *opinion*. All right, I'll steal the M.D.s' thunder right out from under them, and agree with them. It *isn't* a controlled study, no. I want to make it perfectly clear that I have not been able as yet to finish up the extremely complicated experiments that are necessary to statistically *prove* the worth of using vitamin C day in and day out for continuous protection against all colds.

I admit then that I don't have nearly as strong, scientifically satisfactory proof of this particular one of vitamin C's powers as I do of its abilities as a *treatment* for already established colds, or for its value as a one-shot protection against a specific visible contact. Furthermore, I myself will bring up a further flaw in my own reasoning that hasn't even occurred to most of the people who don't want to believe that vitamin C really has. any cold-preventing powers. It's this: most of the letters I get are *nice* letters; they say nice things, such as vitamin C *does* work, yes, Doctor, you're right. People aren't so ready to put uncomplimentary or disagreeing type arguments in writing and then mail them to you. So you can't count on your mail to give you the truth.

Nevertheless, the reports I've received from all over the country are just too overwhelming to deny, and that's because there's one very interesting thing about them: while not a single person who sends me a report on what his school or group is experiencing with vitamin C and colds knows exactly what anybody else is telling me, when you look over these reports here's what you find:

> (1) In general, the greater the routine daily dose of C used at a school, at least from 250 mg. up to the 1000 mg. level, the higher is the reported estimate of the reduction in colds compared to the school's past (before-vitamin C) experience.
>
> (2) If the total daily dose happens to be split into at least *two* portions, *A.M.* and *P.M.,* at a particular school

(and is at least 500 mg.), that school usually estimates a greater success in reducing the number of colds than does another school using the *same* size dose but giving it all at once.

(3) The larger the group of students taking the vitamin C at a school, the larger, though sometimes only slightly, is the estimated apparent reduction in the number of colds suffered by the school.

Since these reports are completely independent of each other, and none of them knows what the others are saying, there's an extremely strong suggestion that some basic truth is operating underneath all this, and that basic truth is not likely to be anything but that vitamin C, when taken on a routine day to day basis in sufficient amount, *does* work to cut down the number of colds caught by a *group* of at least so many persons.

So while there is no guarantee that by taking regular daily vitamin C any one specific individual will positively note a marked decrease in the number of colds he catches, still a person has a pretty good chance for improving his record. And this chance of success is fairly closely related to the size of the dose of vitamin C he takes routinely, and very definitely related to his faithfulness in taking it.

Question: What dosage of vitamin C do you recommend for year-round protection against colds?

Answer: Based on experience with my own patients, and seconded by the physicians and the general public who have written me from many different places, I feel that for an adult a daily dose of 250 or 500 mg. is both useful and perfectly safe. (Children under 80 pounds: 250 mg.) Since individuals do differ in some degree in their response to vitamin C (as they do at least slightly in every other detail of the workings of their body) there is no way to say in advance which of these two recommendations will be sufficient for any one person, that is enough to do the trick for *you* in particular. If you decide to try 500, or find that you need it, split it into 250 mg. in the morning and 250 at suppertime. (It's hardly worth splitting a 250 mg. total daily dose; in fact, that much may be better taken all at once in the morning, before you face people for the day.) I think we can safely say that 100 mg. a day usually won't do the trick, and that a continuing

1000 mg. (one full gram) may be too close to favoring an unfortunate intestinal bacterial flora for many people. My best advice to you at this point is for you to regularly take 250 or 500 mg. daily, except during the summer months. This much vitamin C is surely all to the good and very little to the bad. You can raise it up for brief periods (several days) when the risk of catching a cold is great or a questionable symptom starts giving you a hint.

Question: Are you telling us that you're *not* recommending that we take enough vitamin C on a regular basis to absolutely guarantee that we won't catch *any* cold?

Answer: I do not believe it is in your best interests to aim for a total and complete avoidance of all colds by a *high near-continuous* daily dosage of vitamin C. It seems wiser to me for you to take the moderate routine dosages specified, which are quite likely to reduce to some degree the number of expected colds (and probably also to lighten the severity of those colds that do develop) and then for you to increase vitamin C all the way to treatment levels on some necessary occasions.

Question: Aren't there people who haven't had a single cold in five or even ten years, where that was solely due to their having taken a lot more vitamin C than 250 or 500 mg. a day?

Answer: Yes, there are some people who have had that experience, but I frankly don't like the amounts of vitamin C that most of them took to do it—amounts usually in the range of three grams (3000 mg.) daily, or even five to ten grams every day. That's a lot of vitamin C. I must tell you that much personal experience, and a deal of thinking about what has happened over a long time, have brought me both more admiration *and* more caution about vitamin C. Anyway, some of my own patients demonstrate that colds can be almost totally avoided with considerably less vitamin C than the three to ten gram daily levels we have just mentioned.

Vitamin C at a level like three grams a day, and most particularly at five to ten grams must be considered a "medicine," rather than a "vitamin." It still remains a good general rule that you should not take *any* medicine any longer than you have to, or in any greater dosage than you must. These rules of moderation still hold. Medicines usually have undesirable side effects, especially given time to show them. Vitamin C in medicine amounts and given time also has—or at least may have for some people—its own undesirable side effects. These include (1) disturbance of the intestinal bacterial flora, and (2) acidification of the urine (which in some instances is undesirable). There may well be other unpleasant results on some people. Remember that we're talking here about how much vitamin C is safe for us to take *over long periods;* that's the key point, long periods. We daren't take the same dosages of a medicine over an extended length of time, say three or six months, or two years, as we may dare to take over only short stretches of three days, or 10 or 12 days.

We can't always claim that whatever nature does "naturally" is necessarily the best for us on every occasion, and therefore *we* oughtn't to do anything different, nor can we assuredly make the argument that "if God had wanted us to have a continuous high level of vitamin C in our blood stream he'd have seen to it that we had it," *but* on the other hand a physician is taking his chances— and chances on his patient—if he insists on going against nature's standards for any lengthy period.

Question: And are you also saying that you don't think we should take vitamin C the full year around either, even in small doses?

Answer: I see little value in your taking even preventive vitamin C during the summer months. I think if you're going to take it at all on a near-continuous basis, you should limit it to the "cold season." In New England, for example, the cold season starts in early September as soon as the schools open. I'd suggest you start taking vitamin C on August 15, two weeks before school starts, to build up a level, and then continue it through the next nine and a half months until June 1. An even less lengthy vitamin C season such as December 1 to May 1 will do you most of the good the longer one would.

Question: But what about the so-called "summer" cold? Isn't it true that colds that you do catch in the summer often seem to be quite "strong" ones? Why should this be, and if it's true, why oughtn't we to be taking preventive vitamin C in the summer too?

Answer: For one thing a summertime cold has a very good chance of catching you with your interferon defenses completely down, since you've likely had no cold for a long time. For another, everything is pretty much stacked against colds in the summer—the sunlight, the outdoor life, the fresh foods, the closed schools—so that any virus that can make it against such odds is liable to be one corker of a bug.

However, I as a physician have to view things from the broad view. I'm responsible for a *lot* of people, not just one or two. Summer colds may be bad sometimes, but they're relatively *scarce.* From the point of view of the *group,* we have very little to gain by taking vitamin C during the summer (New England: June 1-August 15), and I feel we should cut it out completely, at least in tablet medicine form. (Fresh fruits and vegetables? Of course, certainly.) This will give our intestinal flora a break from the continuous pressure of medicine vitamin C. For the same reason, once you've just had a cold, no matter when that is, winter or summer, and whether you used vitamin C to *treat* it or not, you should consider cutting down your regular preventive vitamin C somewhat during the following weeks of your earned immunity, unless you're taking only a low 250 mg. anyway.

DETERMINING THE DOSAGE LEVEL FOR YEAR-ROUND PROTECTION FROM COLDS: AN ILLUSTRATIVE CASE

I think it may tie things together a little better if I were to tell you about an actual case I had recently.

A mother asked me what I would recommend for her ten year-old daughter who always seemed to have her colds go on and become complicated by bronchitis (which means the infection has involved the "bronchi," or breathing tubes which carry air to your lungs). She wanted to know how much vitamin C should be used routinely, what size tablets should be given, and when.

After determining that this little girl had no blameable local reason in her nose or throat for these special bronchitis complications, nothing we might have corrected like heavily infected tonsils, for example, and after I made sure that the child was generally in good health I agreed that here was an ideal case for the preventing of colds, if we could carry it out successfully.

Our little patient weighed a good 80 pounds, which is not as much as an adult, but with the danger of lung-tube infection at every cold I wanted her to get enough vitamin C so that her chances of avoiding all colds would be pretty good. So I settled on our trying one cold season on a daily total of 500 mg. for her, one 250 tablet in the morning (before she'd face her schoolmates), the other at 2:30 P.M. when she had just gotten home from school. I cautioned the mother that the first six weeks of vitamin C we were trying wouldn't mean too much, but after that we could expect results. If this schedule did the trick, I said we'd use it again next year, beginning August 15. If it didn't, we'd start the next cold season with a 750 mg. total (one tab at breakfast, lunch, and supper). I said we wouldn't proceed to a 750 mg. daily total unless we'd proved by one season, or a good piece of one, that 500 mg. wasn't sufficient. I also advised the mother that since she was convinced that every single cold brought bronchitis with it, we should be prepared to take special measures if a cold slipped by us and developed. We'd give the child a sizable dose of semi-long-acting penicillin no later than the second day of her cold, and again on the fourth day. (To physicians: 450,000 units, paren-teral.) This penicillin would be given by *needle* after a sensitivity test, because we wanted to make very certain it would get a chance to work.

If, based on past experience, you're certain that some bacterial complication will develop upon the base of the (virus) cold, the proper way to handle this complication is to take measures to stop it *before* it develops. This is not in any way the same as "giving a shot of penicillin for a cold." (That means a plain cold where you *don't* expect a bacterial complication.) But giving penicillin in a situation like we've outlined here *is* striking a blow for *prevention*, of course, and that's always preferable to *treatment*. We try to prevent even the basic cold by routine, moderate-dose vitamin C. If the cold gets past this defense, we decide whether or not to *treat* it with vitamin C. If you're an adult, and good at the treatment, then yes, by all means use vitamin C. If it's a small child, recognize your difficulties with vitamin C *treatment*. But whether you treat the developing cold with vitamin C or not, and whether it's a child or a grown-up, if you have reason to expect a complication you must start treating for it *in advance* (as I did by the penicillin injection) *unless* the cold is being very well controlled indeed. Of course, you'll need your doctor for this. If an *unexpected* complication develops—it *won't*, of course, if this is a well-treated-with-vitamin-C-case—then

get that surprise complication treated with antibiotics. Don't just
take it sitting down.

THERE IS A LOT MORE TO PROTECTING YOURSELF
FROM CATCHING A COLD THAN JUST VITAMIN C

There is quite a bit of evidence that if you take a very large
amount of vitamin C regularly every day of your life it is going to
be nearly impossible for you to catch a cold *ever*, no matter what
the circumstances are. Even if you make a terrible mistake, such as
finding yourself unceremoniously dumped into ten degree pond
water as your punishment for skating on too-thin ice, not even a
chilling shock like that can bring forth a cold if you're on five
grams of vitamin C daily—and if you get pulled out in time. (If
you don't get roped and laddered out within ten minutes you
won't have to worry about the cold one way or the other.)

If you are taking huge amounts of vitamin C daily—three
grams, five grams, *ten* grams, and there are people who are doing
that—neither sudden chilling shock nor less serious oversights on
your part are going to make a particle of difference. You'll never
get a cold. I call taking this much vitamin C solely for *preventive*
purposes a very *big* precaution, to differentiate it from the kind of
"little" precaution we'll be getting to very shortly. And it *is* a
tremendous proof of the great power of vitamin C that you can
actually subject your body to insults that would ordinarily greatly
favor the outbreak of a cold, and yet still not get one *if* you've
been on a continuous five grams a day of the vitamin.

But this ten grams a day immunity to colds is too great a
price to pay for most people, in my considered opinion. And only
if you are "paying the price" by risking taking these tremendous
amounts of vitamin C day in and day out can you afford to
completely ignore and just forget about the many little precautions that can help you so very much to avoid catching a cold
most of the time. Since I don't think it's best for you to take all
that vitamin C on any regular basis (remember I *do* think it is safe
for only 10 to 12 days as *treatment*, not prevention) then we will
have to go ahead and review the good many other things besides
vitamin C in *huge* doses that will help to keep you from catching a
cold. What are these little precautions?

PRECAUTIONS THAT WILL GREATLY CUT DOWN YOUR CHANCES OF CATCHING A COLD

Of course, we're not including the treatment schedule of a 10-12 day course of vitamin C, because here we're talking only about *prevention.*

(1) Vitamin C in *reasonable* regular (preventive) dosage for every member of the family. (250-500, even 750, possibly in a few cases 1000 mg. daily)

(2) Vitamin C in against-a-particular-contact (interceptor) dosage (a two-dose set of 600-750 mg. each)

(3) Physically avoid every obvious cold you possibly can (Turn and run from every sneeze or cough, even if it isn't considered "democratic" to do so. Daddy sleeps on the sun porch if the kids bring home a cold from school. "Nurse"-mother: treat yourself with vitamin C if you catch the cold.)

(4) Avoid the drying out of your breathing surfaces, the mucous membrane linings of the inside of your nose and throat. (Artificial indoor heat is the prime cause of this; use a humidifier.)

(5) Keep yourself in good general health. (Don't let yourself get "run down.")

(6) Avoid fatigue, keep yourself thoroughly rested always.

(7) Don't try to lose weight during the "cold season."

All the rest of these precautions are "avoids," relating to "exposure." ("Exposure" is one of those rather vague words everybody may *think* he knows the meaning of, but when you get right down to having to act on it you have to know precisely what is meant. For your purposes "exposure" means avoiding the specific things mentioned in items 8, 9, 10, and 11 of this list):

(8) Avoid any sudden temperature changes.

(9) Avoid drafts, wet feet, dampness.

(10) Avoid chilling, especially for extended periods. (Get yourself back to warm as soon as you get home; the quickest way is a hot bath in the tub, not a shower.)

(11) Avoid breathing very cold air. (It will "burn" your vocal cords and open them to easy infection.)

For the same reason as number 11 be careful not to yell in a loud voice for very long in very cold weather. In the very coldest air wear a breathing mask over your face and mouth. You can get one at the drugstore. It will raise the temperature in your breathing passages up to a safe, non-"burning" level even if you're breathing through your mouth. If you don't have a mask, at least keep your mouth shut while breathing in cold weather. This will force you to take air in only through your nose, which has very remarkable abilities to warm up cold air almost instantaneously and in only a few inches of space. Your nose will also "humidify" (that is, moisten) the air in the seconds it has it as the air passes through on its way to your lungs. This is why your nose "runs" in cold air. It's producing extra moisture to wet the air you're breathing. A really marvelous, but little understood and even less appreciated piece of equipment, the nose. Air taken in through the mouth is hardly warmed and hardly moistened by comparison.

A little aside while we're on face masks. You'll notice my suggestion for your wearing them is for warming up the coldest air as you breathe it in. Sometimes in Japan you will see people wearing face masks right in the street. This is sometimes a courtesy to keep you from catching their colds, and this *is* probably worthwhile to you as a prospective victim, but it would be still better if the colds stayed at home. As for *your* wearing a face mask *before* you have a cold to keep from catching one, I don't believe it's worth the bother, even if you wouldn't be embarrassed to wear one. (Face masks worn by doctors and nurses in operating rooms are intended primarily to keep the *doctors' and nurses'* germs out of the operation, rather than the other way around.)

Being careful about these last items, numbers 8-11, that make up the picture of "exposure" may sound to you very much like some of those admonitions they used to give you about colds and which you knew very well weren't worth much and were only being suggested to you because there was nothing that really helped. The fact is, however, that every one of these listed hazards genuinely does make it more likely that you will catch and develop a cold, the danger of them is *not* just unfounded old wives' tales. It's true, though, that paying attention to them in the past usually *didn't* keep you from catching a cold anyway. So you may be wondering why we're trundling these old chestnuts out again at this time. I'll tell you why. It's because *now* paying attention to these things *does* make a difference. Now, if you'll use vitamin C in reasonable, daily preventive doses, that is, if you'll follow the number 1 on our list of little precautions, it really makes a difference if you watch out for items 8 through 11. (Items 4, 5, and 6 also make more difference now with vitamin C than they used to, too.)

If you carefully follow all the eleven precautions on our precautions list, you're going to get very few colds, and you're going to be taking only a negligible risk with the amount of vitamin C you're taking to do it.

It is true, though, that a regular preventive dose of vitamin C that will ordinarily do very well to protect you from catching most colds, say a dose of 500 mg. daily (split two ways) still may let you down once in a great while if all the circumstances fit together just right, or rather, just "wrong." Suppose all the following were to be able to hit you at one and the same time: (1) your *not* having had any recent cold to give you at least a tail end of immunity, (2) a heavy dose of sneeze from a "strong," active cold, (3) no interceptor dose of vitamin C handy to take, (4) a deep chill, (5) a marked drying of your throat, (6) something already in your stomach that would effectively have downed the value of your regular daily protective dose of vitamin C (not necessarily yogurt). Be unlucky enough—or careless enough—to get all those blows put together against you at once, and you may miss up and develop a cold in spite of your faithful daily preventive dose of C. I say "may" because the common cold is so persnickety that with all of those things against you, you still may escape. If you lose out, of course you will still be able to successfully *treat* your "bad luck" or "error," as the case may be, if you care to. And the large doses of vitamin C you will have to fall back on to do this will be safely limited to no more than 12 days at any one stretch—the standard treatment schedule.

The *more* vitamin C you take on any regular, continuing basis, the "sloppier" you can get away with being about following these little precautions we have discussed, but the greater the risk you will be taking with these larger amounts of vitamin C. This applies in a gradual way to perhaps five grams of vitamin C a day, at which point you'll have almost absolute protection from colds, precautions followed or not, but this, in my opinion, is at too great a cost in possible undesirable side effects from this much vitamin C on any continuing basis. In general, I feel that the younger you are, and the less scientific training you've had—if any at all—the more caution you should show about taking any larger doses of vitamin C than I have been willing to wholeheartedly recommend to you in this book. On the other hand, if a person has already had some experience of his own with taking vitamin C, he may well have developed the necessary judgment and perspective to perhaps come to a different conclusion about what may be best in his own particular case. And if you are an older person, it is only fair to keep in mind that a senior citizen's body just does not operate quite as efficiently as a younger person's may, so that what may seem to be a higher dose of vitamin C may not really be so high for *him*.

Of course, your own physician can always be counted on to advise you.

We should perhaps say a few more words concerning several of the little precautions on our list.

Drying of the Mucous Membranes and Its Effect on Your Catching Colds

I myself am indebted to Dr. Joseph Lubart of New York, who has kept on stressing the importance of keeping one's respiratory membranes (surface linings of the nose and throat) normally moist if you want to avoid catching all possible colds. These cell surfaces are supposed to be slightly wet, they work best this way and they resist viruses best this way. These layers of cells lining the breathing passages are the body's first line of defense for the nose and throat, just as the skin is the first defense on the more outside areas of the body's surface. These mucous membranes can do a lot to keep "bugs" (viruses) from making an entrance, but they don't work nearly as well at it if they're too dry, or if they're colder than they should be. Very cold air is also drier than usual, and when you breathe it the drying effect may very well be more dangerous than is the measurably cooled *temperature* of the tissues at the time. If you want vitamin C to be able to protect you from catching most of the colds you run into, and to be able to successfully suppress the few that get past you, you have to give it a little reasonable help here and there. Take care of your mucous membranes by not letting them get dried out, and they'll take care of *you* by being able to exclude a lot of bugs in the first place, which is ever so much better than having to eject these undesirable little creatures from your body at a greater expense later on.

There was a period where for over two years I had to continue to face up to the fact that there had still been one glaring, unexplained flaw in the otherwise perfect record of my success with vitamin C's being able to beautifully control every developed cold without exception. You see, there *had* been one exception. A cold had once broken out on me at the very time when I had been regularly taking a fairly substantial dose of vitamin C for months. I could not understand this. It spoiled the whole picture of vitamin C and colds that had been slowly building up for me. Only very much later was I able to recognize that on the evening in question I had sat fully within the arch of a great flaming colonial fireplace for hours, and in so doing had dried my breathing surfaces. Which brings us to the principal factor that is responsible for the drying out of our breathing membranes in these days. It is the heating of our houses in winter, perhaps the *overheating,* because now we do insist on having our houses much warmer than they were a century ago. Winter air is drier than summer air, ordinarily, and when it comes indoors and is heated it becomes drier still. When we breathe it in we cannot help but dry our noses and throat surfaces to some extent. However, we can counteract this rather nicely by using a simple little humidifier. This need not be an expensive piece of furniture with a lot of moving parts turning inside it. An inexpensive one is merely a plastic dish with an electric element to form steam, and costs less than $10. It uses about the same current as a light bulb of moderate brightness. Keep one in any room you use a lot, especially the bedroom, and on the coldest nights let it puff away for a few hours in the evening. It need not run all the time.

The Effect of Sudden Temperature Changes on Your Susceptibility to Catching Colds

Let's talk a little about sudden temperature changes and how they may dispose you to a cold. This is one of the connections that has been noted for a very long time already, and it's a true one. Like the other hazards that can make you more liable to breaking out with the virus, this particular change in the weather doesn't *always* produce a cold, of course, because there are so many other factors that have to be allowed to throw their two cents' worth into the final decision as to whether you, J. Jones, will be favored with a cold at this time or whether you will not. But, J. Jones, just don't jump yourself aboard the nearest plane and jet down to Florida on a February 1st to get yourself an oh-so-welcome break from the icy grip of a New England winter, that is, don't do it and then think you're going to get away with it scot-free. Your chances of getting a cold, or two of them (one on the way back, too) are *greater* than if you'd just stayed up here with us poor folks who can't afford the trip. Of course, part of the reason for your troubles is that you sealed your body into a poorly ventilated vessel along with scores of other dangerous, virus-carrying specimens of the human animal. But another part of your seemingly special susceptibility to cold viruses at this time clearly relates to the abrupt change of climate that can result from swift air transportation. Any relatively fast, rather unexpected shift in your external environment, the climate you live in, is liable to work changes in your internal environment, too. One such change, there can be no doubt, is in your relative resistance to cold viruses. Such changes as do occur seem to be your *disadvantage*. Going toward a warmer, "nicer" place is not necessarily any less shocking to your body than your moving in an unfavorable, colder direction. Of course you need not personally move your own body quickly from one climate to another to respond to this sort of change in the weather; it also applies if a changed *climate* moves *itself* rapidly in on *you,* and you haven't moved from your spot. That's how the laziness of spring fever hits you. But if you're the one who stays still and lets the changing climate do the moving, you at least won't be running the extra risk of that close confinement with your fellow man in the belly of the big bird.

WHAT HAPPENS IF YOU HAVEN'T HAD A COLD
FOR THREE OR FOUR YEARS

Now we can leave our precautions list and talk about something completely pleasant for once. I found out with my patients during the course of our experiments that if you haven't suffered through an ordinary cold, that is, haven't gone through a full-blown one for some three to four years, you become somewhat less likely to get a cold at all than you were before that long stretch of cold-free time. To earn this sort of reward it wasn't necessary for you to have successfully avoided even *catching* any cold for a solid four year period. It was only necessary that you *either* avoided catching colds *or* that you rapidly cooled off every one of them that you did show up with, cooled it off with vitamin C.

After several years of no colds to speak of—as a result of their increasing understanding combined with the ministrations of vitamin C—some of my patients seemed to have changed so that they didn't pick up colds as quickly as they had before. Now, these people were *not* taking vitamin C as a continuing preventive, *that* wasn't what accounted for their now-lessened susceptibility to colds. At first I thought it was just that these people had had such marvelous training in the art of avoiding colds, and had learned their lessons so well that they were unconsciously now doing all the "right" things, or possibly not doing all the "wrong" ones. As a matter of fact, almost everybody who stayed with me did show the effects of his greatly increased understanding of the workings of the common cold "monster," and by the end most everyone was catching fewer colds than he had caught in the past, whether he took preventive vitamin C in either of the two preventive ways (regular daily, or just-at-a-specific-contact) or whether he didn't take it at all. But there was more to it than this; it seemed pretty definite that if your body had become relatively "unfamiliar" with cold symptoms because you hadn't had any for several years, at least not any fully developed ones, then you didn't seem to react to viruses quite as openly as you had before. This applied both to the ease with which you accepted viruses (you didn't catch cold as easily now) and it also applied to the degree of your response to them once caught—the symptoms of your developed colds were often milder than they had been in earlier years.

You can often boil all that last down to just this: cut down the number of colds you catch at all and cut down on the severity of the ones that did get you—you do this by brains and vitamin C—and you may get not only *this* "money in the bank," this "principal," you may actually earn yourself some "interest" too—a somewhat lessened susceptibility to colds, an advantage that'll hold for at least a while into the future, maybe quite a while. Even if it doesn't last, or if I'm all wrong about this end of it, still you'll have learned a lot by now, and *that* will certainly stand you in good stead from here on.

Addendum

A Note to Physician-Readers
on the Possible Mechanism of Action
of Vitamin C Against the Common Cold

Many physicians have written me after reading my original professional report asking me what I felt was the mechanism of vitamin C's successful action against colds. The following is a copy of the answer I have sent to these correspondents:

The mechanism of vitamin C's action against colds was not commented upon in the report, because the study provided no valid evidence on a microbiological level. None of the basic physiological presumptions out of which the picture to follow has been constructed originated with me, of course. I merely was to pick them up and try to fit them to my observations, largely through the process of logic. I never have and do not now grant to this application of them any inevitable certainty. Indeed, too great a confidence in the infallibility of similar speculations was, in the past, the very feature which blocked some investigators from moving on to the higher dosages which would quickly have shown them what ascorbic acid really can accomplish for the common cold. With this disclaimer of any necessary certitude, let us go on. As far as the power to suppress visible symptomatology is concerned, two possibilities suggest themselves, neither of which has to be a correct one, of course. Common cold symptoms are by and large expressions of the inflammatory reaction (thus, for example, hoarseness results when plasma and cells exude into the vocal cords). Perhaps vitamin C works by limiting the magnitude of the inflammatory reaction. One of "C's" presumed activities is

185

a decrease in capillary permeability. Capillary walls rendered less permeable could not pass as much inflammatory fluid into the tissues as otherwise, even if the antigens "requesting" this response were to be present in their normal battle numbers. The need for closely continuing administration of the drug to keep symptomatology in check dovetails well with this explanation. But another and different one is by no means ruled out. Vitamin C may work solely by seeing to it that no very great inflammation has to be called for in the first place. This is exactly what would obtain if the offending viruses were to be cheated of their rightful multiplication: an inferred activity of vitamin C which may or may not be different from "decrease in capillary permeability," namely the power to make individual tissue cell membranes less penetrable by viruses, could be responsible. Each time the intruders would seek to break from a conquested tissue cell and to violate a fresh one they would find their passage disputed in both of these directions. Now, as for prophylaxis of colds rather than suppression, it also might reside in this same cell intransigence to virus perforation. The initial invaders would find themselves forced to face up only to stubborn cell walls. Unable to start off their intracellular colonies in sufficient force they would be foiled for this one battle at least.

Analysis of those instances where vitamin C's performance as either prophylaxis or suppressive has left something to be desired commonly reveals an evident lapse of anti-respiratory-infection discipline such as one of the following: either the victim has been subjected to an imposing example of too-low respiratory humidity, or had suffered himself to remain chilled for an extended period, or the treatment ascorbic acid itself had lost cogency through oxidation, or was taken in too small dosage. A not-likely-to-be-thought-of source for a dosage effectively too small is the presence in the intestine of an absorptive agent such as yogurt that traps part of the ascorbic acid. There is a possible common denominator on the microbiological level to all of these mishaps: a relatively eased pierceability of the respiratory cell walls. In these "failure" cases so many organisms got an intracellular foothold that proportionately they overwhelmed vitamin C's then-current membrane blocking capabilities.

Suppose vitamin C really has no capability to keep colds viruses from their customary replication, then are we not taking something of a risk when we elect to use it to limit the amplitude of nature's inflammatory response to this *not*-diminished force of organisms? Well, my perhaps ill-judged readiness to so promptly write off as expendable a benison with so good an "image" as "the inflammatory reaction" may proceed from my observation of what irremediable havoc that process may inflict upon the human eye, admittedly with its need for unimpaired transparency something of a special case. But, as stated above, flouting the possible importance of inflammation has seemed to have been without serious punishment in the common cold. If the viruses responsible for the affection are really not lethally alarming ones, and if the ordinary consequences of their assault can fairly be classed as little more than annoying, then it may be entirely fitting for us to feel a degree of freedom about hindering the evolvement of the inflammatory base upon which secondary, more grave dangers sometimes thrive, even if it be at the cost of a slight retardation in accomplished immunity.

Why won't vitamin C restrain the inflammatory reaction and hence the symptomatology if it be started only on the third or fourth day of a cold? Because the edema and cellular elements already on the spot by then will take days to clear up even if new exudation can be kept from joining them, and also because by this time you will be fighting an amplified army of the little monsters.

Index